REAL BABY FOOD

EASY, ALL-NATURAL RECIPES FOR YOUR BABY & TODDLER

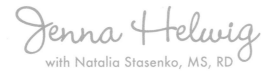

Jenna Helwig

with Natalia Stasenko, MS, RD

To Rosa—
my sweet, brave,
funny girl.

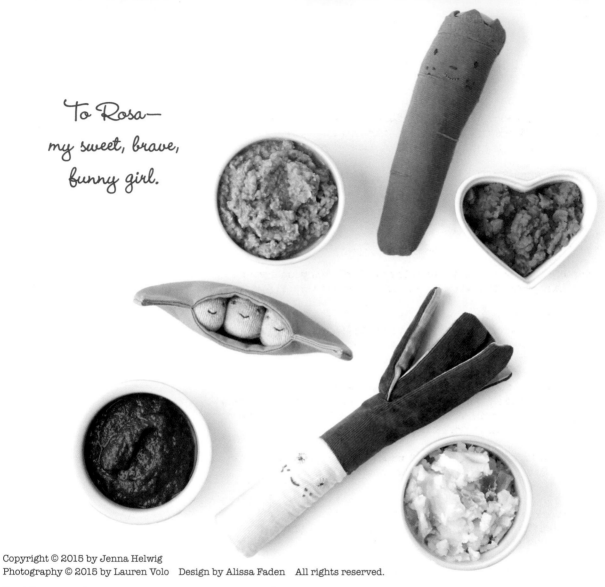

For information about permission to reproduce selections from this book, write to Permissions,
Houghton Mifflin Harcourt Publishing Company, 215 Park Avenue South, New York, New York 10003.

www.hmhco.com

Library of Congress Cataloging-in-Publication Data
Helwig, Jenna.
Real baby food : easy, all-natural recipes for your baby and toddler / by Jenna Helwig ; with Natalia Stasenko, MS, RD
pages cm
ISBN 978-0-544-46495-7 (paperback) — ISBN 978-0-544-46496-4 (ebook)
1. Infants—Nutrition—Popular works. 2. Toddlers—Nutrition—Popular works. 3. Cooking (Natural foods)—Popular works.
I. Title.RJ216.H3575 2015   641.5'6222—dc23   2015005794

Printed in the United States of America   DOC 10 9 8 7 6 5 4 3 2

Acknowledgments

Thank you to Sharon Bowers, my delightful agent who happens to be a terrific writer herself. Receiving every one of your emails is a pleasure, and I am indebted to you for your guidance throughout each step of this process.

I am so grateful to Adam Kowit. I couldn't have asked for a more thoughtful or considerate editor. It has been a pleasure crafting this book together. And a big thank you to the rest of the excellent team at Houghton Mifflin Harcourt, including Rebecca Liss, Claire Holzman, Michelle Bonanno, Brad Parsons, Jessica Gilo, Molly Aronica, Helen Seachrist, Melissa Lotfy, and Alissa Faden for the gorgeous design of *Real Baby Food*.

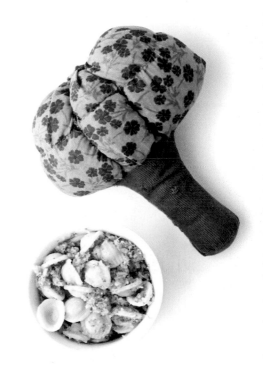

Lauren Volo, your photos are exactly what I hoped for. Thank you for your generous eye, calm presence, and the warm vibe you created on set.

Sharon Bowers once said that food stylists are "magic." I couldn't agree more, especially when it comes to the lovely and talented Mariana Velasquez. Prop stylists belong in the magic category, too, especially Alix Winsby who got the book's look and feel just right. Thank you both.

I couldn't ask for a better collaborator than Natalia Stasenko. Your deep knowledge about feeding and nutrition makes this book better in every way. And the fact that you worked so hard on this project amidst the birth of your third child and a trans-Atlantic move continues to amaze me.

Thank you to Suzy Scherr for sharing your creative, toddler-pleasing recipes, and thank you to Nicole Page for your friendship and sage advice.

I am grateful for the support of my colleagues at *Parents,* especially Dana Points and Chandra Turner. Thank you also to my longtime friend and colleague Steve Engel and his incomparable wife Heidi Reavis, plus all of my Rosaberry chefs and clients.

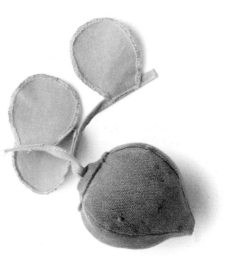

With love and gratitude to my dear friends Danielle Wilkie, Allison Graham, and Felicity Rowe.

Of course, thank you to Linda and Andy Helwig (for everything, really). Their unflagging enthusiasm for this book manifested itself in last-minute grocery runs, movie dates with Rosa, and the taste testing of many, many recipes. Thanks also to David and China Helwig, especially for hosting me in your Seattle home and giving me the opportunity to observe the adorable Cole and Tasha's eating habits at close range.

And finally, thank you to Dave and Rosa. You sacrificed your summer weekends to this project, cheered me on, and gamely tried dish after dish. Without you at the table it wouldn't matter what was served. I love you.

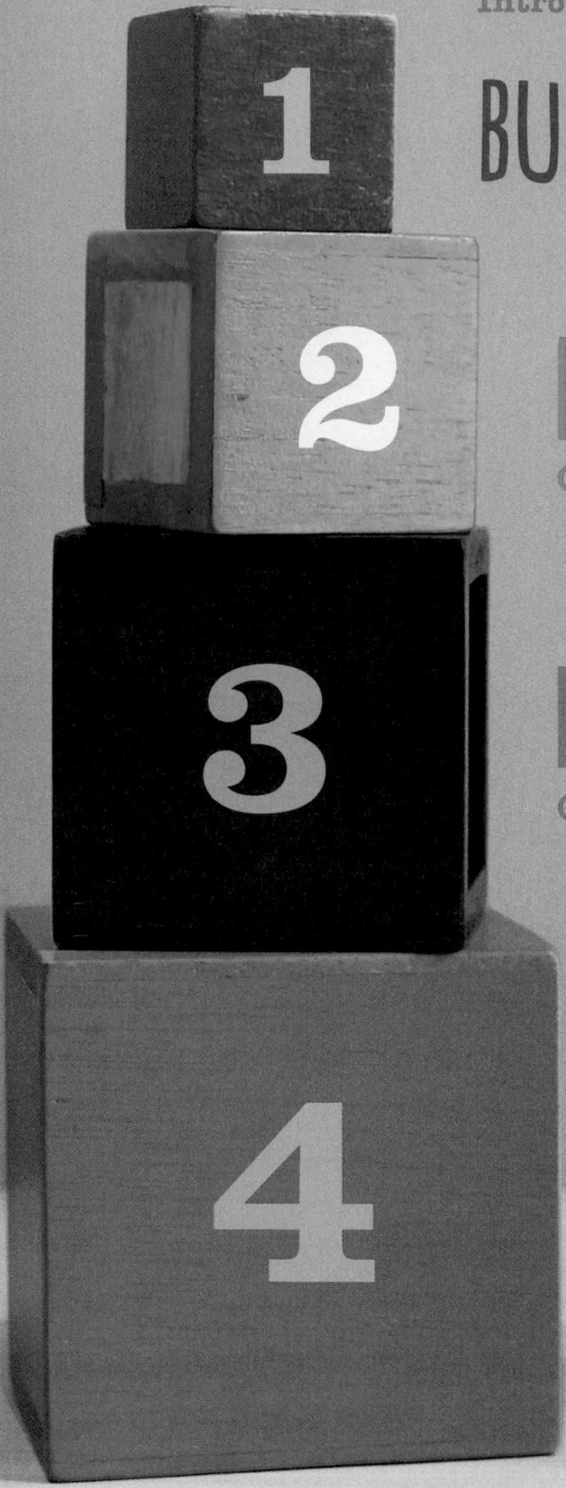
1
2
3
4

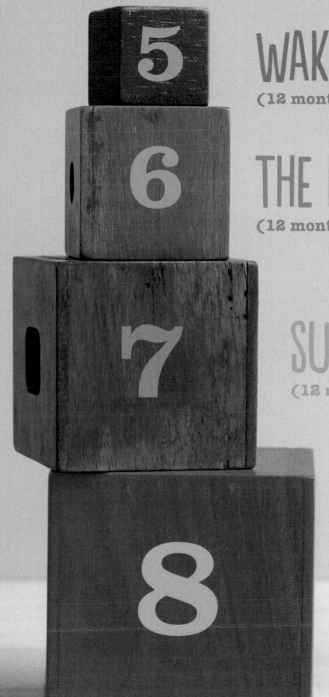

INTRODUCTION

When my daughter started eating solid food, I knew one thing: offering Rosa a grayish purée of green beans or an odorous mash of processed chicken and rice was out of the question. I wouldn't touch that stuff. (I could barely stomach opening the jar!) So why should she? Plus, I wanted my daughter to be omnivorous. Bland, jarred baby food seemed like a step in the wrong direction.

Instead, I started making large batches of my own purées and freezing most of it, so I had baby food on hand whenever we needed it. I cooked and mashed apples from the farmers' market and broccoli from the grocery store. I puréed cooked ground chicken and mashed up roasted cod. I kept a few jars of packaged baby food on hand for emergencies, and used store-bought, iron-fortified baby cereal, but for the most part it wasn't hard to make sure my daughter was able to eat homemade food on a daily basis.

I came to believe in homemade baby and toddler food so much that I launched a business helping parents learn how to make their own. I worked with moms and dads who were eager to get their little one off to a good culinary start, but unsure of where to begin. A few years later I became Food Editor at *Parents* magazine, and I was convinced all over again. There is a *hunger* (truly!) for knowledge about DIY baby food and a growing understanding of how important the first months of eating are in a child's development. Parents want to perform this simple, natural task for their children, and thankfully, with just a little bit of kitchen savvy, it's completely achievable.

That's where this book comes in. *Real Baby Food* will give you the know-how and the inspiration to make your own fresh, healthy, tempting meals for your child from the moment she takes her first bite of solid food to the time she is happily ensconced in a booster seat at the family dinner table. The recipes come from my own experience cooking for Rosa, as well as years of teaching classes and feeding clients' kids. From Broccoli-Apple Swirl (page 53), to Rosemary Roasted Pears (page 70), to Saucy Meatball Sliders (page 190), baby and toddler food doesn't have to be boring. In fact, it can and should be delicious, a tasty primer for a child's developing palate.

Making your own baby food is also easy. I'll show you a simple method to ensure you

---

A RECENT STUDY HAS SHOWN THAT THE MORE FLAVORS BABIES ARE EXPOSED TO BEFORE AGE ONE, THE MORE LIKELY THEY ARE TO ENJOY FRUITS AND VEGETABLES AS OLDER CHILDREN.

---

always have healthy food on hand, with little to no cooking on a daily basis. Preparing homemade baby food truly can fit into anyone's schedule.

WHY SHOULD YOU MAKE YOUR OWN BABY FOOD?

I believe in the power of homemade food at every stage of life. It is healthier, cheaper, fresher, and often better tasting than anything that comes from a box, can, bag, or delivery container. But we're all busy people, especially new parents. Why should moms and dads make their own baby food when there are so many options—organic even!—available at the supermarket? Here's why: your best shot at raising a child who loves to eat nourishing, real food is to cook it yourself and eat together from the very earliest days. And there's more!

- Homemade food is fresher, meaning fewer nutrients will be lost as the ingredients travel from farm to table.

- Homemade food is less processed. Should beef stew really be shelf-stable?

- Homemade food can be less expensive: You will save money by making food in batches.

- The ingredients are under your control. Does your baby love peas? Add them to chicken stew. Do you want organic or non-GMO foods? Your call.

- The food contains no preservatives, and there is no added sugar, salt, or oil beyond what you choose to include.

- The food tastes better. Feeding toddlers, especially, can be a challenge. It's a no-brainer that they're more likely to eat a meal that doesn't taste like it came from a can or box.

- By feeding your baby fresh, flavorful meals you are training his taste buds, helping him become accustomed to the variety of flavors that await him.

- While your baby is in taste-training, you are in kitchen-training. Whether you cook regularly already or are just learning, making your own baby and toddler food will start you on a journey in the kitchen that will hopefully continue as your family grows. Making homemade food will benefit your baby's and your health for many years to come.

- For many parents there is also something profoundly satisfying about not outsourcing this important part of their child's growth. Making your own food is a generous way of showing your love.

HOW TO USE THIS BOOK

Real Baby Food will be your guide, from your baby's first bite of solid food through her toddler years, and my hope is you will use many of the recipes long beyond that. Chapter one, Building Blocks, covers all of the information you need to know as your baby starts solids: when to start, with what food, and how much your baby should eat on a daily basis. I also cover what cooking equipment you'll need, special ingredient considerations, and ways you can help ensure your baby grows into a happy, willing eater.

In chapter two, First Tastes begins with recipes for 10 Starter Purées, excellent choices for your baby's first foods. The chapter continues with other single-ingredient purées, and a few basic blends. Turn to chapter three, New Flavors, once your baby has tried and is comfortable with a variety of the simple purées in First Tastes. At this point she's primed to enjoy more blends, and probably ready for a chunkier texture as well. That said, the recipes in both chapters can be puréed as much or as little as you like, depending on your baby's comfort with lumpy food.

Chapter four features fun Finger Foods, perfect for babies around eight months and older. While you should feed your baby simple finger foods as soon as he starts solids, once he has more of a handle on chewing, the recipes in this chapter will become your mainstays. Next, it's toddler time! Once your baby is a year old he is ready to move on to the Breakfast, Lunch, Snacks, and Dinner chapters in the second half of this book. Many of these recipes are sized for sharing with the whole family.

In addition to easy-to-make recipes, *Real Baby Food* addresses numerous nutrition and feeding topics. To ensure this information was top-notch, I worked with Natalia Stasenko, MS, RD, a pediatric dietitian and the mother of three young girls. She also contributed a nutritional analysis of each recipe so you will know exactly what you're feeding your child. Natalia has a passion for feeding children well, and it shows throughout the book.

ABOUT THE RECIPE ICONS

 30 Minutes or Less – These meals are ready to serve in under half an hour.

 Freezer-Friendly – These recipes are ideal for making ahead and freezing, or for freezing leftovers for a future meal. Unless otherwise noted in the recipe, dishes with this icon hold up well in the freezer for up to three months. And unless the recipe suggests otherwise, for best results defrost frozen food overnight in the fridge or thaw in the microwave. Never let food defrost on the countertop for more than an hour.

 Construction Zone – Empowering little ones to choose what they eat makes it more likely that they'll try new foods. So dishes marked with this symbol can be separated into components so toddlers (and everyone else) can assemble their own meal at the table. This might be as simple as choosing whether to top Chicken Soba Soup (page 214) with sliced scallions, or as elaborate as assembling a complete dinner, as in the Fajita Salad (page 192).

A NOTE ON NUTRITION

Each recipe in this book features nutritional information, but it's helpful to know how much of each nutrient your child needs on a daily basis. Remember these numbers are just ballparks. Don't panic if your little one isn't meeting these exact benchmarks every day of the week.

	6-12 months	1-2 years	2-3 years
Calories	600–900	1000–1400	1000–1400
Protein	11 grams	13 grams	13 grams
Fiber	N/A	19 grams	19 grams
Calcium	260 mg	700 mg	700 mg
Iron	11 mg	7 mg	7 mg
Potassium	700 mg	3000 mg	3000 mg
Vitamin C	50 mg	15 mg	15 mg
Vitamin A	2000 IU	2000 IU	2000 IU

Keep in mind that the recipe serving sizes are quite small, especially for babies just starting solids (only two tablespoons!), so few of the nutrient numbers will be very high. Also, remember that your baby is still getting a large proportion of his nutrition from breast milk or formula.

chapter one

BUILDING BLOCKS

Introducing Solids and Beyond

When you're about to feed your baby solid food for the first time, it's important to be familiar with the most recent official recommendations from groups like the American Academy of Pediatrics (AAP) and the World Health Organization (WHO). But it's even more critical to know your child and to be flexible when it comes to the timing and choice of solid food.

WHEN TO START

The formal guidelines by the AAP and WHO recommend exclusive breastfeeding for the first six months of life. Starting solids before four months has been related to increased risk of obesity and future food allergies, while delaying solids beyond six months may lead to a deficit of certain nutrients in the diet, such as iron and zinc in breastfed babies, and delays in oral-motor function.

We recommend starting solids between four and six months of age and closer to six months if possible. When determining whether it is time to start the solid food adventure, be guided by your baby's eating skills and body control. Here are some of the signs that your baby may be ready for solids:

- Your baby sits up with support. Not all babies can sit unsupported at six months. A couple of cushions on both sides of the high chair may help her be more comfortable. But if your baby is still not able to sit straight, consider waiting a week or two.

- Your baby has neck and head control and can hold them still.

- Your baby gives you cues. Is he is interested in the food you are eating? Trying to grab your spoon?

- Your baby can close her lips over a spoon.

- Your baby loses the thrust instinct and his tongue no longer pushes out food from his mouth.

- Your baby keeps food in her mouth and swallows it.

HOW TO START

Finally, your baby is ready! You prepared some yummy food and cannot wait to introduce him to all the amazing flavors. Just a few reminders before that very first spoonful ends up in your baby's mouth:

- Make sure your baby is sitting straight. A high chair works better than a recliner or baby bouncer. This way, your baby will be more comfortable when mastering this new way of eating.

- Put some food on your baby's lips first to let him experience the texture and get curious about what's coming.

- Always wait for your baby to pay attention before starting to feed. Do not put anything in a child's mouth without her permission. It may be extremely tempting to just sneak a spoonful of food into her mouth while she is distracted, but that strategy may quickly lead to increased pressure at mealtimes. Many babies react to pressure by eating smaller amounts and being less interested in feeding.

- Let your child decide how much food he wants and whether he wants to eat. Some babies want to eat a lot of solid foods from the first feeding, while others want a teaspoon or two, and some are not interested at all. At this age solid foods are not likely to contribute significant nutrition to your baby's diet and even a small amount is an important exposure. Do not feel like he needs to finish a whole serving and do not feel pressured to serve a "typical" portion size. At the end, it is your baby who determines the amount he wants to eat at each feeding.

> CONSIDER THE FIRST FEW MONTHS OF STARTING SOLIDS AS A "TASTE-TRAINING" PERIOD AND SET A GOAL OF EXPOSING YOUR BABY TO AS MANY FLAVORS AS POSSIBLE.

- Stop feeding immediately when your baby is no longer showing interest. Most babies make it clear that the meal is over by being more distracted by their surroundings, turning their heads away, and closing their lips. By pushing your baby to eat even a little more you may make meals unpleasant for both of you and potentially interfere with your baby's ability to self-regulate.

- Try including the baby in family meals, even if it's just "playing" with a few Cheerios, or perhaps eating tiny bites of the food you are having. This will help him feel included in the family meal and learn to like the foods that you are enjoying.

WHAT TO SERVE

By the time your baby is six months old, her stores of iron and zinc are diminishing and she also needs a source of vitamin C in her diet, so it's important to provide her with good sources of these nutrients. Until recently, conventional feeding advice has been to start with a baby rice cereal and move on to vegetables, fruit, and other foods. And while purchased baby rice cereal is not a bad choice because of its high iron content and low likelihood of allergenic response, the recent recommendation from the American Academy of Pediatrics is to explore other nutritious options as well, such as vegetables, fruit, eggs, meats, and other cereals. All of these make excellent first foods.

Your baby may not like the flavor or texture of some foods at first, but don't stop serving them to your child. Studies show that the more food experiences babies have in the first two years of life, the more varied a diet they eat as schoolchildren. And while starting with fruit probably doesn't prevent babies from liking vegetables later, introduction of solids is a perfect time to allow babies to experience the flavor of green vegetables and other foods with slightly bitter flavors. Your little one may not like it at first, but if you are consistent and keep offering green vegetables daily, your patience will pay off—now, and when many of your child's buddies hit the picky eating stage around age two.

HOW TO SERVE YOUR BABY'S FIRST MEALS

Start with one-ingredient purées, so if your baby has an allergic reaction you'll immediately know the culprit. If you are introducing a new food, offer it in the morning to have time to observe your baby for signs of allergic reaction during the day. If possible, wait at least 24 to 48 hours before introducing each new food,

since it often takes that long for an allergic reaction to manifest.

Try to plan solid meals when your baby is neither starving nor too full. If you are formula feeding, offer solids a little earlier than the regular feeding time and "top up" with the bottle after that. However, if your hungry baby gets easily frustrated when offered food in this novel fashion, experiment with giving a little bit of formula first and letting your baby finish it after the solid meal. If you are breastfeeding, you can offer solids after you breastfeed so that your baby can get all the goodness of the less-filling breast milk.

Your baby may take some time to learn how to handle the totally new texture of solid foods. Keep the first purées very thin, just a little thicker than the milk or formula your baby is drinking. As your baby learns to master this first challenging texture, it is time to serve thicker purées and purées with lumps. Research shows that babies who are transitioned to more challenging textures as soon as they are ready are less likely to have feeding problems later in life. For most babies, the transition to lumpy purées happens within the first few weeks of starting solids. As soon as he has no trouble handling a certain texture, it is time for an upgrade!

WHAT TO DRINK

Babies get most of the water they need from breast milk or formula when they are starting solids. However, it is a good idea to introduce

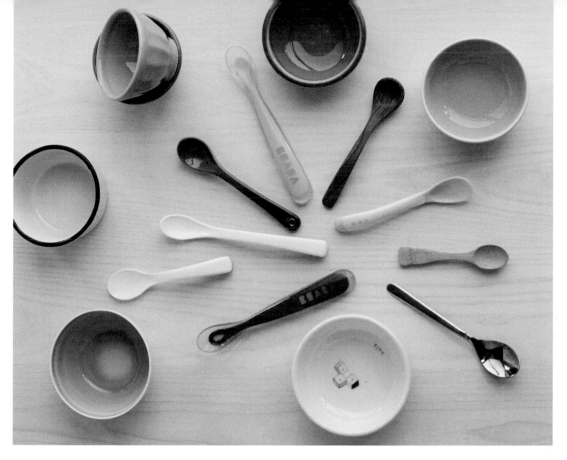

a sippy cup with a little water (1–2 oz.) at mealtimes when your baby is first eating solid foods to allow her to practice using it. At the age of eight to ten months most babies can enjoy drinking their water and formula from a cup with a straw. After 12 months of age, most babies can drink their water and cow's milk from an open cup with a little help, and they can be weaned off a bottle gradually.

WHAT'S NEXT?

Babies should practice with simple finger foods (see page 96) from the earliest days of starting solids, but by the time they are about

eight months old they will likely be ready for more complex flavors and textures. At this stage you should incorporate both finger foods and spoon-feeding into each meal on a relatively equal basis, provided your baby has enough motor control for this. (Unless of course your baby refuses to eat from a spoon. In that case, just up the finger foods.)

By the time your baby is about a year old he will probably be ready to eat regular meals with the family. The recipes in the second half of this book are ideal for your toddler both in terms of taste, texture, and nutrition, and will likely make everyone else in the family very happy as well.

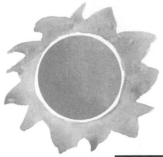

Portion Sizes for Babies

Babies aren't one-size-fits-all, but this chart will give you a general sense of appropriate portion sizes and how to break up a baby's daily meals. Since some babies need more food and some babies need less, serving amounts are approximate. Intake from one day to another also fluctuates.

	4 TO 6 MONTHS	6 TO 8 MONTHS	8 TO 10 MONTHS	10 TO 12 MONTHS
FIRST THING IN THE MORNING	Breast milk on demand or 6–7 oz. of formula	Breast milk on demand or 6–7 oz. of formula	Breast milk on demand or 6 oz. of formula	Breast milk on demand or 6 oz. of formula
BREAKFAST	1–2 tablespoons of cereal/grains 1–2 tablespoons of fruit or vegetable	2–4 tablespoons of cereal/grains 2–4 tablespoons of fruit or vegetable	4–6 tablespoons of cereal/grains 2–4 tablespoons of fruit or vegetable	4–6 tablespoons of cereal/grains 3–4 tablespoons of fruit or vegetable
MIDMORNING	Breast milk on demand or 6–7 oz. of formula	Breast milk on demand or 6–7 oz. of formula	Breast milk on demand or 6 oz. of formula	½ serving of dairy 3–4 tablespoons of fruit or vegetable
LUNCH	1–2 tablespoons of cereal/grains 1–2 tablespoons of fruit or vegetable OR Breast milk on demand or 6–7 oz. of formula	1 serving of grain 2–4 tablespoons of fruit or vegetable Breast milk on demand or 6–7 oz. of formula	2–4 tablespoons of protein 2–4 tablespoons of fruit or vegetable 1 serving of grain Breast milk on demand or 6 oz. of formula	2–4 tablespoons of protein 3–4 tablespoons of fruit or vegetable 1 serving of grain Breast milk on demand or 6 oz. of formula

1 serving of grain = ½ cup cereal or cooked rice, quinoa, pasta, or couscous, ½ slice bread or 2 crackers. Choose brown rice, whole grains, and whole-wheat pasta about half the time.

1 serving of dairy = 1 cup (8 oz.) of full-fat yogurt or 1.5 oz. of full-fat cheese. Cow's milk is not recommended for infants under 12 months, but cheese and yogurt are fine.

	4 TO 6 MONTHS	6 TO 8 MONTHS	8 TO 10 MONTHS	10 TO 12 MONTHS
MIDAFTER-NOON	Breast milk on demand or 6-7 oz. of formula	Breast milk on demand or 6-7 oz. of formula OR ½ serving of dairy	2-4 tablespoons of fruit or vegetable 1 serving of grain OR ½ serving of dairy	3-4 tablespoons of fruit or vegetable 1 serving of grain OR ½ serving of dairy
DINNER	Breast milk on demand or 6-7 oz. of formula	1-3 tablespoons of protein 2-4 tablespoons of fruit or vegetable 1 serving of grain	2-4 tablespoons of protein 2-4 tablespoons of fruit or vegetable 1 serving of grain	2-4 tablespoons of protein 3-4 tablespoons of fruit or vegetable 1 serving of grain
BEFORE BED	Breast milk on demand or 6-7 oz. of formula	Breast milk on demand or 6-7 oz. of formula	Breast milk on demand or 6 oz. of formula	Breast milk on demand or 6 oz. of formula

Portion Sizes for Toddlers

Just like babies, toddlers' feeding needs aren't set in stone. Your child will vary from the one next door, who will vary from the one across the street. These portion sizes are just meant as a general guide.

AGES 1 TO 2	AGES 2 TO 3
2 cups of dairy per day	2-2½ cups of dairy per day
2 cups of fruits/vegetables per day	3 cups of fruits and vegetables per day
2 oz. of protein per day	3-4 oz. of protein per day
3 servings of grains per day	4 servings of grain per day

Kitchen Tools

In its essence, making baby food is really quite simple. All you need to do is cook some food until it's soft (although you don't always even need to cook it!), and purée or mash it until it's smooth enough for your baby to eat at her stage of development. How you cook and how you mash are the variables.

Generally, I like to cook a baby's food by either roasting or steaming, depending on the ingredient. Unlike boiling, both of these methods help proteins, fruits, and veggies retain their inherent nutrients. To purée or mash, different tools give different results. A basic blender makes for the smoothest, most velvety purées, although sometimes it's a challenge to blend dense ingredients like squash. A food processor makes quick work of any vegetable, but depending on the ingredient, it can be difficult to get a perfectly smooth purée. Since both of these machines have different strengths I recommend one or the other in most baby food recipes, but generally, you can default to a simple blender. That said, both of these machines are worthwhile investments since you will use them to cook for your family for years to come.

An immersion blender is another handy option, as you can place it directly into a bowl or pot to purée food. This also saves some dishwashing time (always a good thing). While an immersion blender can make for a smooth purée, it can be a challenge to remove every single lump, so I find this appliance the most convenient for recipes when your baby is a bit older and ready for food with more texture. Finally, an inexpensive ricer or food mill is ideal for mashing potatoes, both now and at countless Thanksgivings down the road.

As your baby gets more proficient at chewing, probably around eight to ten months, a fork will be the only mashing tool required.

Here is all the equipment you'll need to make wholesome, nutritious food for your child:

To prep:

Large cutting board	Measuring cups (both wet and dry)
Sharp chef's knife	Measuring spoons
Small paring knife	

To cook:

Steaming basket	Rimmed baking sheet
Medium saucepan and large pot with lids	Parchment paper and foil

---

To purée or mash (choose one or more):

Standard blender	Food mill or ricer
Food processor	Immersion blender

To store:

Ice cube trays	Zip-top freezer bags or other airtight containers

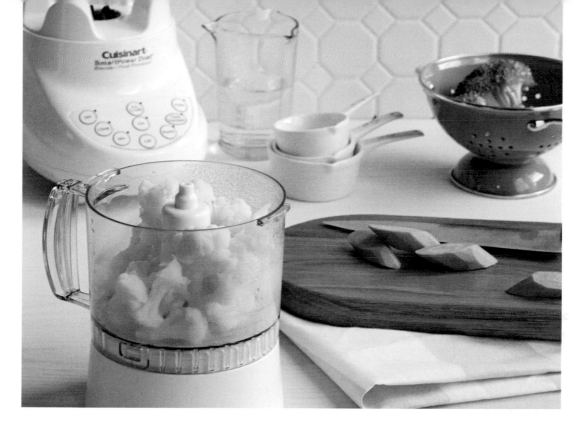

Ingredients

While cooking for a baby or toddler isn't radically different than cooking for any other human, there are important things to keep in mind regarding specific ingredients and food groups.

Breast Milk & Formula: Whether your baby drinks breast milk or formula, this food will continue to comprise a hefty part of his diet until his first birthday. See the portion chart on page 9, but know that formula needs vary. Some babies prefer to drink formula in smaller amounts more frequently, while others are satisfied with bigger amounts less often. Make sure to stay attuned to your baby's hunger/satiety cues when bottle feeding to allow him to drink just as much as he is hungry for. Generally, after introduction of solids, most babies need around 32 ounces of formula a day, divided into four to five feedings. Around the age of eight to ten months, when solid snacks are introduced, the amount of formula your baby needs will go down to 24 to 28 ounces, divided into three to five feedings.

Breast milk or formula also comes in handy when serving purées to younger babies. Any time a purée or cereal is too thick, simply thin it with a little breast milk or formula.

Dairy: Cow's milk is not recommended for infants under 12 months, but cheese and yogurt are fine. At the age of 12 months babies can be transitioned to 16 ounces of full-fat cow's milk daily, instead of formula or breast milk. If your child eats yogurt and cheese, in addition to drinking cow's milk, limit all dairy intake to the equivalent of 16 ounces or two servings of dairy.

Until age two babies should consume full-fat dairy, such as milk and yogurt. After that you can switch to reduced or low-fat.

Sugar and Other Sweeteners: Avoid most, if not all, added sugars for babies under 12 months. Learning to love less-sweet foods will be a boon as your child enters a sugar-laden world. And avoid honey and corn syrup completely before 12 months of age, since botulism spores can contaminate these sweet ingredients.

Salt: Before 12 months there is no need to salt your baby's food; their little bodies don't require much sodium. After 12 months, use salt judiciously, but know that a little salt can go a long way to bring out the flavor in food, especially in proteins and veggies. When cooking I prefer coarse, kosher salt.

Herbs & Spices: Baby food doesn't have to be—and in fact, shouldn't be—bland. Experiment with herbs and spices to jazz up simple purées and blends. As long as you don't make a meal too spicy (hot), your baby will likely enjoy the flavor. Each recipe in First Tastes includes a Flavor Kick suggestion, but feel free to try out different combinations.

Pantry Items: Having a well-stocked pantry and condiments shelf in the fridge will make cooking on a regular basis much easier. Here is a basic list of the foods I have kept on hand since my daughter's earliest days of eating solids:

- Canned beans (look for cans without BPA in the lining)
- Canned or boxed tomatoes
- Whole-wheat and regular pasta
- Quinoa
- Brown and white rice
- Whole-wheat crackers
- Oats
- Panko bread crumbs
- Maple syrup
- Honey
- Dijon mustard
- Mayonnaise
- Olive oil
- Canola oil
- Balsamic vinegar
- Red and white wine vinegar
- Chicken and vegetable broth
- Nuts
- Dried fruit
- Whole-wheat and all-purpose flour
- White and brown sugar
- Baking powder and baking soda
- Salt

Freezer-Full: Frozen vegetables such as chopped spinach, broccoli, corn, and peas are super convenient and just as healthy as fresh. Make sure to stock plenty of frozen fruit as well. I keep raspberries, blueberries, mangoes, and bananas (that I peel, chop, and freeze myself) on hand at all times.

Iron-rich Foods: Be iron-savvy. Iron-rich foods like meat, fish, poultry, egg yolks, beans, and green vegetables should be served to children at least twice daily. Iron from animal sources (heme iron) is absorbed better than iron from plant sources (non-heme iron). The American Academy of Pediatrics recommends feeding iron-fortified cereal to toddlers until the age of at least 18 months. If you are raising a vegetarian baby see page 88 for a list of non-meat sources of iron.

Should You Go Organic? Whether you're making all of your own baby food or supplementing with some purchased food, you'll need to decide if you want to spend the extra money for organic produce or meals. This is a personal decision based on priorities and budget.

As you weigh the pros and cons, keep in mind that conventionally-produced fruits and vegetables harbor a higher concentration of pesticides compared with organic food. While most research has shown that the pesticide level in conventional food is safe, many new parents choose to err on the side of caution and buy organic, especially since chemical pesticides accumulate in higher levels in small children.

One option is to buy organic versions of the fruits and veggies that typically harbor the highest amount of pesticides. The Environmental Working Group (ewg.org) makes this easy for us by tracking the "cleanest" and "dirtiest" fruits and veggies in terms of pesticide load.

Another alternative is to strive to buy organic the food that your child eats the most frequently. In my household that was cow's milk (once my daughter was 12 months old) and eggs. Since she consumed so much of these two foods it made good sense to me to buy organic even though it was more expensive. Whenever possible I also buy organic dairy, meat, and poultry, or versions that are raised without antibiotics or artificial growth hormones.

Remember that the most important thing, though, is to feed your family lots and lots of fruits, veggies, and healthy proteins whether they are organic or not. The benefits of these nutritious foods far outweigh any of the negatives. So don't feel guilty if springing for organic isn't in your budget.

Cooking in Bulk

One of the reasons DIYing baby food is much less daunting than it may seem is because it's so easy to cook in large quantities. Make a batch of sweet potatoes or applesauce and you'll have enough purée for 16 servings for babies just starting solids and eight servings for older babies. Simply keep two to three days' worth in the fridge and then freeze the rest in ice cube trays. Once the purées are frozen, pop them out of the trays and store them in large zip-top bags or other containers. If you make three different purées on Sunday, and the following week you make three more, you'll have almost 100 servings of baby food to mix and match over the course of the coming weeks. With just one or two exceptions, all of the recipes in First Tastes and New Flavors make enough for several servings.

AS A GENERAL RULE, BABY FOOD (OR PRETTY MUCH ANY FOOD) KEEPS IN THE REFRIGERATOR FOR UP TO THREE DAYS AND IN THE FREEZER FOR UP TO THREE MONTHS.

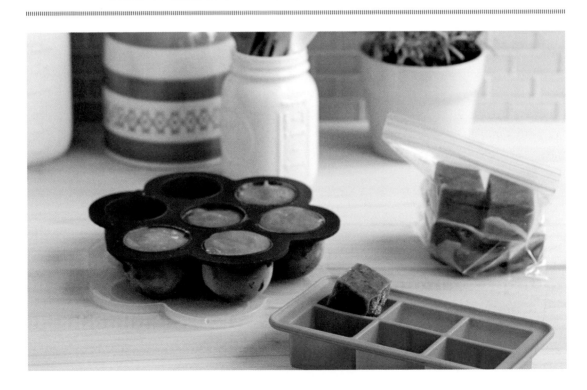

10 RULES FOR PREPARING HOMEMADE BABY FOOD

1 Practice safe food handling practices. Always wash your hands before cooking and after handling raw meat, eggs, or poultry. Avoid cross-contamination by thoroughly washing your cutting board and knife after chopping raw proteins.

2 Before steaming, roasting, or poaching food, cut it into similarly-sized chunks so the pieces cook at about the same rate.

3 Be careful when puréeing hot food in a blender. Let the food cool slightly, then remove the plastic insert from the blender top, and cover with a towel before blending. This will reduce the pressure inside of the blender and make it less likely that your kitchen ends up a spattered mess.

4 Add water (or breast milk or formula) by the tablespoonful to the blender or food processor to help the purée blend smoothly. Scrape down the sides frequently.

5 Store baby food in the fridge for up to three days and in the freezer for up to three months.

6 Be sure to label containers of baby food, especially when freezing, with the name and date. I use masking tape and a permanent marker.

7 Thaw baby food overnight in the refrigerator. Food for your baby should never sit at room temperature for longer than an hour.

8 If you reheat food in the microwave, stir it thoroughly before serving to disperse any pockets of heat.

9 Avoid adding salt and anything beyond a small amount of sugar to your baby's food for the first 12 months.

10 Make your baby food in bulk. Freeze it into small portion sizes so you'll always have food at the ready. You'll build up a stockpile of food in the freezer and most days you'll simply be reheating, not cooking.

Baby food keeps beautifully in the freezer for up to three months. Just label the containers or bags with the purée's name and the date you made it. Be sure to freeze the food in ice cube trays or other small portions (2 tablespoons is ideal) so you can defrost a single serving at a time.

To defrost, place the cubes in the refrigerator overnight or gently thaw the purée on the stovetop or in the microwave. Be sure to stir well and test the temperature carefully before feeding your baby. You want the food to be cool, at room temperature, or just warm—never hot.

Raising a Happy Eater

I love to eat—vegetables, burgers, sushi, chocolate, fruit, bread, quinoa, yogurt, you name it. Food is one of the most important elements of my life. I look forward to breakfast, lunch, and dinner every single day. Each meal is an opportunity to taste something delicious, while doing something good for my body. While I didn't expect my daughter to be omnivorous right away, I wanted to give her the gift of loving wholesome, satisfying food.

If you also want to raise children who eat a balanced diet, who don't shriek at the sight of vegetables, who can sit at the table during mealtime with the family, who truly appreciate the pleasures that food has to offer, then making your own food is a powerful first step. As parents, one of our most important roles is to teach our children how to nourish their bodies in a healthy, balanced, and delicious way. If we don't cook for them, and eat with them, it's a much tougher job.

Making your own baby food not only beautifully meets your child's nutritional needs, it also sets her on the path for a lifetime of happy eating. Recent studies have shown that the more flavors babies are introduced to before age two, the more likely they are to eat a plethora of fruits and vegetables as they grow up.

To help you meet that goal, *Real Baby Food* also provides guidance for setting up healthy daily food routines and making decisions about what and when to feed your baby and toddler.

Most parents say they don't want their kids to grow up eating only chicken nuggets, plain pasta, and French fries. In most cases, there is a simple solution: don't feed children chicken nuggets, plain pasta, and French fries. Instead offer them Honey Mustard Chicken (page 200), Pasta with Spinach Pesto (page 105), and Roasted Potatoes (page 212). Feed them

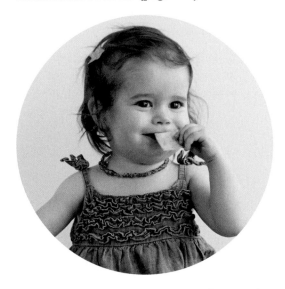

the same foods you eat. Will they always eat it? No. Will there be trying times…trying years even? Possibly. But my message is simple: Don't. Give. Up. Continue cooking for and eating with your children. They will emerge on the other side with a strong lifelong relationship toward healthy food. And armed with recipes and strategies, you will be happier, saner, and calmer around the dinner table.

10 RULES FOR FEEDING YOUR BABY

1 Transfer just a few tablespoons of food into a dish to feed your baby. You'll want to discard whatever he doesn't eat since bacteria from the inside of his mouth will have been transferred via the spoon to the food in the bowl.

2 Watch your baby's cues, and never force him to eat if he doesn't want to. If he closes his mouth or turns his head, just move on.

3 Always supervise your baby and toddler when he's eating. Choking is a real hazard.

4 Start by serving your baby single-food purées. Wait at least one to two days before introducing another food in case there is an allergic reaction.

5 Just because your baby doesn't like a food, don't stop serving it. Babies often need to be exposed to a new food up to 10–15 times before they'll accept it. Try mixing it with a purée you know he enjoys.

6 Aim to introduce your little one to as many new foods as possible in his first 12 months of life. This will help prime his palate and hopefully make him a more adventurous eater later on.

7 Don't stay in the smooth purée stage for too long. Once your baby swallows easily, transition to chunkier meals.

8 To thin a purée, add a little breast milk, formula, or water. To thicken a purée, stir in a little instant baby cereal.

9 A baby's appetite varies from one day to the next—this is normal!

10 Don't be shy about feeding your baby healthy fats such as olive oil, avocado, nut butters, dairy butter, or cheese. And be sure to give children under age two full-fat milk and yogurt. Fat is imperative for growing brains.

Your baby has a lifetime of eating adventures ahead of him. *Real Baby Food* will help you make your child's earliest days at the table (or in the high chair) full of fun, discovery, and good nutrition that will set him on the road to health and happiness.

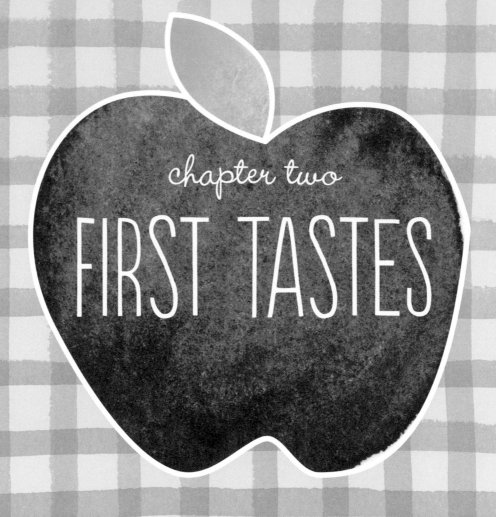

chapter two

FIRST TASTES

SIMPLE PURÉES FOR A WHOLESOME START
(6–8 months)

I started my daughter on solid food when she was just a few days shy of six months old. My plan had been to wait until the half-year mark, but I could tell she was *hungry*. Her little mouth chewed with nothing in it, she watched intensely as my own fork traveled to my mouth, and she tried to grab some of my meal whenever possible. It was clear she was ready for something more substantial than milk, so we eased in to what I hoped would be a healthy, pleasurable eating adventure that would last her whole life. I made two to three purées every weekend, which gave me plenty of stock in the freezer to feed her throughout the week.

Little did I know at the time, but I would look back on those first few months of feeding as Rosa's gastronomic golden age, and you probably will too. During this period, your baby is likely to taste and enjoy more new flavors than ever again, and this is an amazing opportunity to help shape her palate to appreciate fresh, wholesome food.

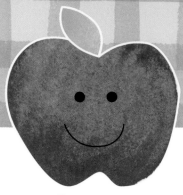

at this stage

Launch your baby's eating career with one of the Top 10 Starter Purées. Feed her just one for a day or two, making sure you don't see any signs of allergic reaction (see page 64). Then move on to another, and then start mixing them.

Since your baby is still getting most of her nutrition from breast milk or formula, don't worry if it seems like she isn't eating very much. But if you find that your baby doesn't like a certain purée, don't give up. Try again in a week or two, or mix it with a purée that you know your baby eats with gusto.

Each starter purée recipe has tips for broadening your baby's culinary horizons. Once you've successfully fed your baby a particular purée, experiment with a Flavor Kick, a dash of herbs, spices, or other concentrated taste. The Purée Playdates section (see page 58) offers blending suggestions to create more complex flavors.

Of course, puréed foods have plenty of applications beyond feeding babies! Age It Up tips offer ideas for transforming purées into grown-up recipes, from blending them into a soup to adding salt and butter for a savory side dish.

During this period add a few simple finger foods to your baby's tray such as Cheerios, cooked beans, or small chunks of soft fruit. See no-recipe-required finger foods, page 96, for more ideas. Chances are your baby won't eat much of these foods yet, but eating with her hands is an important skill to begin practicing.

It's also time to introduce a sippy cup. Serve just a splash of water, breast milk, or formula at each meal and after a few messes your baby will be a pro at drinking—and eating—like a big kid.

SERVING SIZES

Plan on starting your baby with a small serving of just 2 tablespoons. As she starts to eat more over the coming weeks, increase the serving size to ¼ cup. Most of the recipes in this chapter make at least 1½ cups of food, so there is plenty to freeze for future meals.

10 Starter Purées

APPLE

PEAR

POTATO

SWEET POTATO

CAULIFLOWER

RED LENTIL

ZUCCHINI

BUTTERNUT SQUASH

SWEET PEA

GROUND BEEF

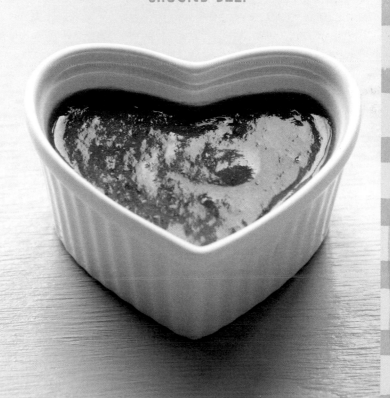

APPLE PURÉE

4 MEDIUM APPLES, PEELED, CORED, AND CUT INTO 1-INCH CHUNKS

Apples were my daughter's first taste of solid food. I'll never forget how her eyes lit up when she tasted this delicious, wholesome purée.

1 In a medium saucepan, bring 2 inches of water to a simmer. Place a steamer basket over the water. Add the apple chunks. Cover and steam until tender, 12 to 15 minutes. Cool slightly.

2 Transfer the apples to a food processor or blender. Process until you get the desired consistency for your baby, adding a tablespoon or more water to the blender if needed to help it blend.

Makes about 2 cups

FLAVOR KICK: Purée with ¼ teaspoon ground ginger.

AGE IT UP: Who doesn't love applesauce? Hold onto this recipe for a perfect lunchbox food as your child grows.

Nutrition per serving (2 tablespoons): 24 calories; 0g protein; 0g fat (0g sat. fat); 6g carbohydrates; 1g fiber; 5g sugars; 1mg sodium; 3mg calcium; 0mg iron; 49mg potassium; 2mg Vitamin C; 26IU Vitamin A

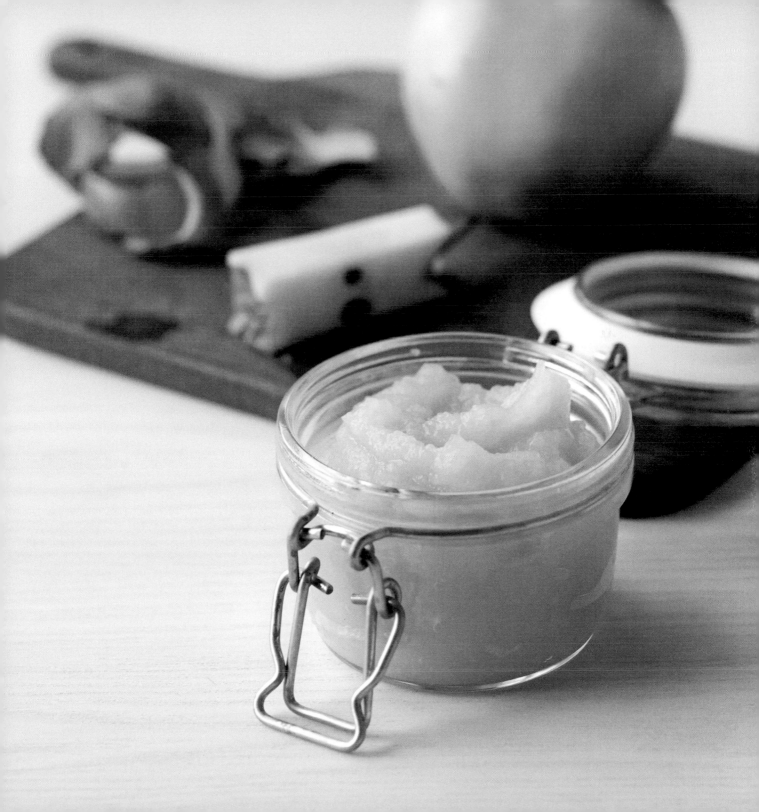

PEAR PURÉE

4 PEARS, PEELED, CORED, AND CUT INTO 1-INCH CHUNKS

Look for ripe Bartlett pears for this sweet baby-pleaser of a purée.

1 In a medium saucepan, bring 2 inches of water to a simmer. Place a steamer basket over the water. Add the chopped pears. Cover and steam until tender, about 8 to 10 minutes. Cool slightly.

2 Transfer the pears to a food processor or blender. Process until you get the desired consistency for your baby, adding a tablespoon or more water if needed to help it blend.

Makes about 2½ cups

FLAVOR KICK: Blend in ⅛ teaspoon cardamom.

Nutrition per serving (2 tablespoons): 20 calories; 0g protein; 0g fat (0g sat. fat); 6g carbohydrates; 1g fiber; 4g sugars; 0mg sodium; 3mg calcium; 0mg iron; 42mg potassium; 2mg Vitamin C; 8IU Vitamin A

10 Starter Purées

POTATO PURÉE

Potatoes often got a bad rap, but they are anti-oxidant-rich and have enough Vitamin C to be nutritionally meaningful. Plus they are a perfect mild food to blend with stronger flavors as your baby's palate progresses. This is one recipe where you want to go low-tech, since a food processor or blender will turn potatoes into a gummy mess. Stick with a ricer (perfect for mashed potatoes) or food mill for a silky purée, or a potato masher for older babies.

2 MEDIUM RUSSET OR YUKON GOLD POTATOES, PEELED AND CUT INTO 1-INCH CHUNKS

1 In a medium saucepan, bring 2 inches of water to a simmer. Place a steamer basket over the water. Add the potato chunks. Cover and steam until tender, about 15 minutes. Cool slightly.

2 Transfer the potatoes to a ricer or food mill to purée, or mash with a potato masher until you get the desired consistency for your baby.

Makes about 2 cups

FLAVOR KICK: Stir in a teaspoon of lemon juice.

Nutrition per serving (2 tablespoons): 18 calories; 0g protein; 0g fat (0g sat. fat); 4g carbohydrates; 0g fiber; 0g sugars; 1mg sodium; 2mg calcium; 0mg iron; 69mg potassium; 2mg Vitamin C; 1IU Vitamin A

SWEET POTATO PURÉE

2 MEDIUM SWEET POTATOES, WELL-SCRUBBED

This is one of the sweetest, smoothest, and healthiest foods you can feed your baby. While you could peel, chop, and steam sweet potatoes, roasting cuts down on prep time and add a delicious, caramelized flavor. Unlike regular potatoes, they blend like a dream in either a food processor or blender.

1 Preheat the oven to 425°F. Line a rimmed baking sheet with aluminum foil.

2 Place the sweet potatoes on the baking sheet and roast for about 45 minutes, or until they are completely tender when pierced with a fork.

3 When the sweet potatoes are cool enough to handle, spoon the flesh out of the skin and into a food processor or blender. Process until you get the desired consistency for your baby, adding a tablespoon or more water to the blender if needed to help it blend.

Makes about 2 cups

FLAVOR KICK: Purée with a ½ teaspoon of ground cumin.

AGE IT UP: Don't forget about this recipe at Thanksgiving, or any fall or winter evening. Add some butter, maple syrup, and a pinch of salt for a scrumptious, seasonal side dish.

Nutrition per serving (2 tablespoons): 14 calories; 0g protein; 0g fat (0g sat. fat); 3g carbohydrates; 1g fiber; 1g sugars; 5mg sodium; 5mg calcium; 0mg iron; 43mg potassium; 2mg Vitamin C; 2971IU Vitamin A

10 Starter Purées
CAULIFLOWER PURÉE

This recipe yields a lot of cauliflower. Luckily, it's an incredibly versatile and healthful purée. Use a bigger pot, 5 quarts if you have it, to accommodate all of the florets. And feel free to include the chopped core and leaves.

1 MEDIUM HEAD CAULIFLOWER, CUT INTO FLORETS

1 In a large pot, bring 2 inches of water to a simmer. Place a steamer basket over the water. Add the cauliflower florets. Cover and steam until tender, 15 to 20 minutes. Cool slightly.

2 Transfer the cauliflower to a food processor or blender, working in batches if necessary. Process until you get the desired consistency for your baby, adding ¼ cup or more water to the blender if needed to help it blend.

Makes about 5 cups

FLAVOR KICK: Add ¾ teaspoon turmeric.

Broccoli Purée: Steam 6 cups broccoli florets (about 1 bunch), until tender, 8 to 10 minutes. Continue with Step 2. Makes about 2 cups.

Carrot Purée: Peel and trim 1 lb. carrots. Chop the thick parts into ½-inch coins and the skinnier parts into 1-inch pieces. Steam until tender, about 10 minutes. Continue wtih Step 2. Makes about 1 cup.

Nutrition per serving (2 tablespoons): 4 calories; 0g protein; 0g fat (0g sat. fat); 1g carbohydrates; 0g fiber; 0g sugars; 4mg sodium; 3mg calcium; 0mg iron; 44mg potassium; 9mg Vitamin C; 0IU Vitamin A

10 Starter Purées

RED LENTIL PURÉE

1 CUP RED LENTILS, RINSED

Full of protein and simple to cook, lentils deserve a prominent spot on your baby's menu of first foods.

1 Bring a medium saucepan of water to a boil. Add the lentils and simmer until tender, stirring occasionally, 12 to 15 minutes. Using a ladle or measuring cup, spoon off and reserve ¼ cup cooking water. Drain the lentils and cool slightly.

2 Transfer the lentils to a blender. Blend until you get the desired consistency for your baby, adding a tablespoon or more of the reserved cooking water if needed to help it blend.

Makes about 1½ cups

FLAVOR KICK: Stir in 2 tablespoons of grated Parmesan cheese.

AGE IT UP: Unsurprisingly, lentil purée easily doubles as lentil soup. Thin it with chicken or vegetable broth, salt to taste, reheat, and serve.

Nutrition per serving (2 tablespoons): 19 calories; 2g protein; 0g fat (0g sat. fat); 3g carbohydrates; 1g fiber; 0g sugars; 0mg sodium; 3mg calcium; 1mg iron; 60mg potassium; 0mg Vitamin C; 0IU Vitamin A

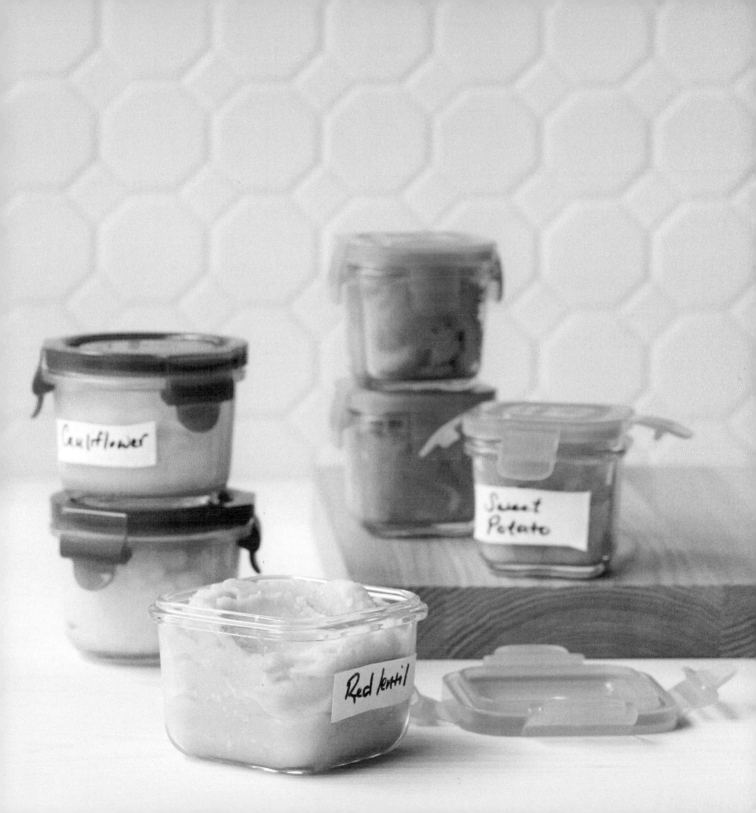

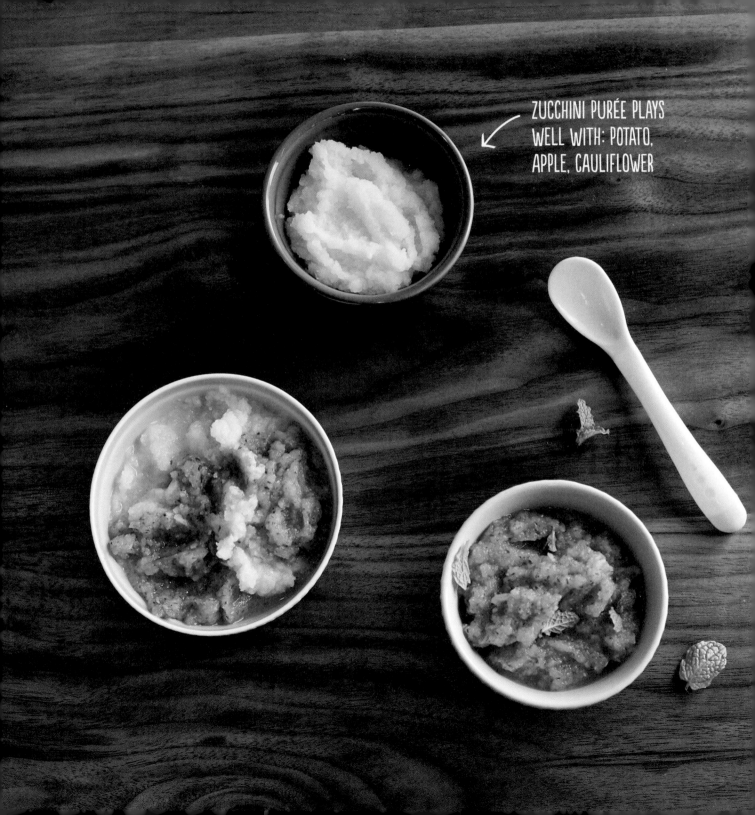

ZUCCHINI PURÉE PLAYS WELL WITH: POTATO, APPLE, CAULIFLOWER

ZUCCHINI PURÉE

There's no need to peel the zucchini for this bright green sauce. A blender makes for the smoothest purée, and because zucchini is so moisture rich, you likely won't need additional water. Yellow summer squash is an easy substitute.

2 MEDIUM ZUCCHINI, CUT INTO 1-INCH CHUNKS

1 In a medium saucepan, bring 2 inches of water to a simmer. Place a steamer basket over the water. Add the zucchini. Cover and steam until tender, about 12 minutes. Cool slightly.

2 Transfer the zucchini to a blender. Blend until you get the desired consistency for your baby, adding a tablespoon or more water if needed to help it blend.

Makes about 2 cups

FLAVOR KICK: Purée with 1 tablespoon chopped mint.

AGE IT UP: This makes a stunningly good cold soup come summer. Refrigerate the purée for at least several hours, add some cream or milk to thin it, salt to taste, and serve in chilled bowls or mugs.

Nutrition per serving (2 tablespoons): 4 calories; 0g protein; 0g fat (0g sat. fat); 1g carbohydrates; 0g fiber; 1g sugars; 2mg sodium; 4mg calcium; 0mg iron; 64mg potassium; 4mg Vitamin C; 49IU Vitamin A

BUTTERNUT SQUASH PURÉE

1 MEDIUM BUTTERNUT SQUASH

The sweet taste of butternut squash is usually an instant hit with babies. This is another vegetable I prefer to roast as opposed to steam, especially since it means no peeling! A food processor will make the quickest work of this purée.

WHOLESOME TIP

Always wash hard fruits and vegetables with soap and water before cutting them, even if you're discarding the peel. This will keep dirt and bacteria on the peel from contaminating your knife, the cutting board, and the cut parts of the produce.

1 Preheat the oven to 425°F. Trim the squash, cut in half lengthwise, and scrape out the seeds with a spoon.

2 Line a rimmed baking sheet with parchment paper. Place the squash halves cut-side down on the baking sheet. Roast until completely tender when pierced with a fork, about 40 minutes. Let cool.

3 When the squash is cool enough to handle, spoon the flesh into a food processor or blender. Process until you get the desired consistency for your baby, adding ¼ cup or more water to the blender (or a little water to the food processor) if needed to help it blend.

Makes about 2½ cups

ALTERNATE COOKING METHOD: Butternut squash also steams beautifully. Peel the squash with a vegetable peeler, halve, scoop out the seeds, and chop. Or buy pre-cut squash.

FLAVOR KICK: Add ¾ teaspoon of ground cinnamon.

Nutrition per serving (2 tablespoons): 25 calories; 1g protein; 0g fat (0g sat. fat); 7g carbohydrates; 1g fiber; 1g sugars; 2mg sodium; 27mg calcium; 0mg iron; 197mg potassium; 12mg Vitamin C; 5953IU Vitamin A

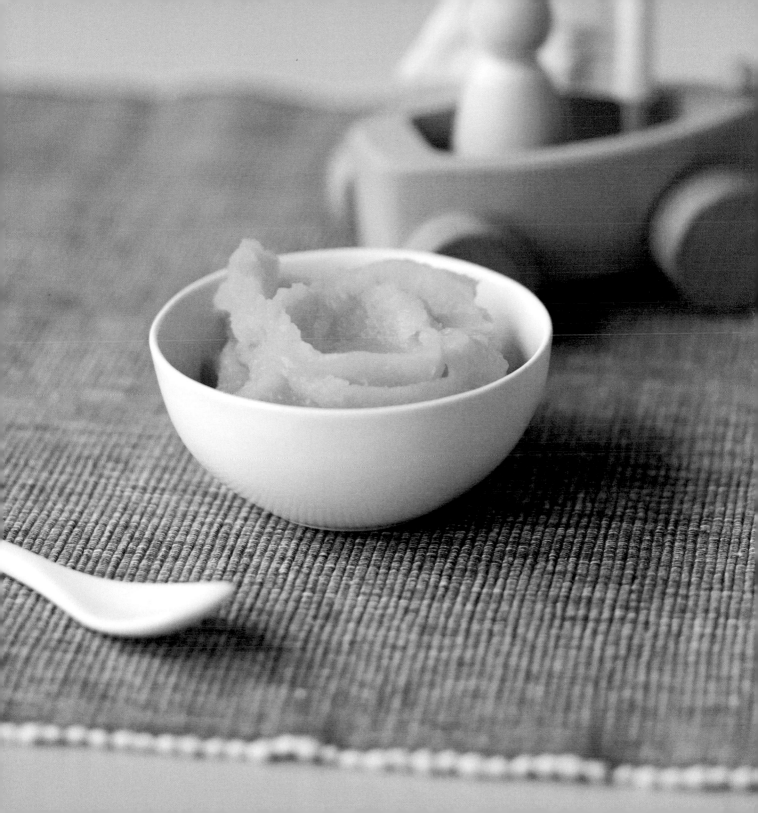

10 Starter Purées

SWEET PEA PURÉE

ONE 10-OZ. PACKAGE
FROZEN PEAS

You can feel good about using frozen peas for this silky, sweet purée. Since they are picked and frozen at the height of freshness, frozen fruits and vegetables are just as nutritious as their fresh counterparts. Be sure to buy frozen produce with no additional ingredients. For a perfectly smooth purée, opt for a blender.

1 Defrost the peas according to package directions. Drain off all but 1 to 2 tablespoons of water.

2 Transfer the peas and water to a blender. Blend until you get the desired consistency for your baby, adding a tablespoon or more water to the blender if needed to help it blend.

Makes about 1½ cups

FLAVOR KICK: Add 1½ teaspoons of chopped fresh basil.

Nutrition per serving (2 tablespoons): 19 calories; 1g protein; 0g fat (0g sat. fat); 3g carbohydrates; 1g fiber; 1g sugars; 1mg sodium; 6mg calcium; 0mg iron; 58mg potassium; 9mg Vitamin C; 181IU Vitamin A

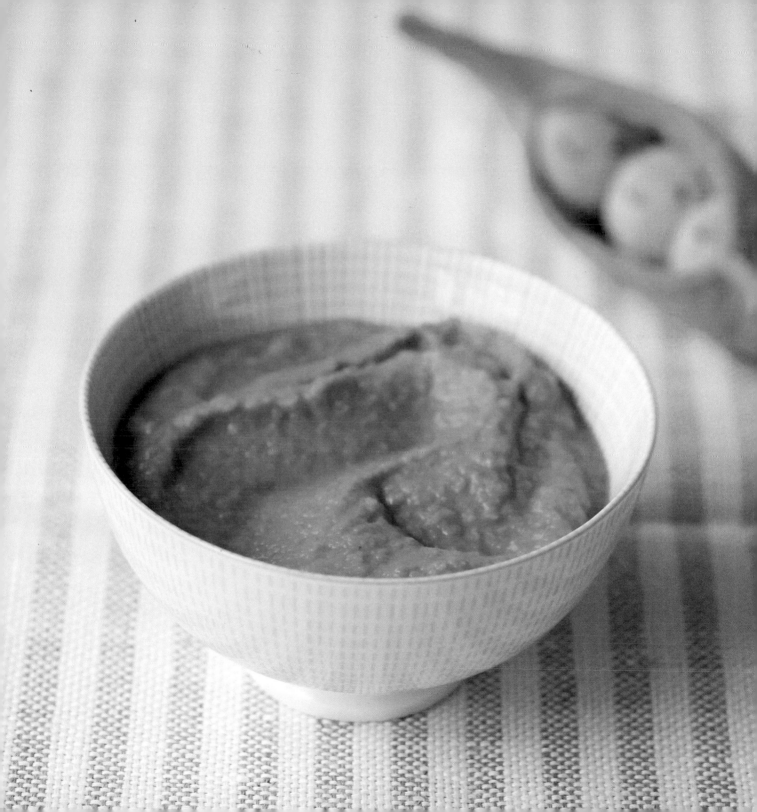

GROUND BEEF PURÉE

1 LB. GROUND BEEF, PREFERABLY ORGANIC

While it may seem unusual to include meat as a first food, protein and iron-rich beef is incredibly healthy for babies. Use the blender for the smoothest texture.

1 Heat a medium-sized skillet over medium-high heat. Add the ground beef and cook until no longer pink, about 7 minutes. Drain and discard fat. Cool slightly.

2 Transfer the beef to a blender. Blend until you get the desired consistency for your baby, adding ¼ cup or more water to the blender if needed to help it blend.

Makes about 1¾ cups

FLAVOR KICK: Blend in a tablespoon of tomato paste.

Lamb Purée: Use ground lamb instead of beef. Makes about 1 cup.

IRON BABY

Babies are born with about six months' worth of iron in their bodies, so as they grow it's important to offer adequate amounts of this critical mineral through food. This is especially important for babies who are nursing since breast milk is low in iron. (Formula is fortified.) Good sources of iron include beef, chicken, beans, peas, green beans, sweet potatoes, and fortified cereals. Between six and twelve months of age babies should eat about 11mg of iron each day.

Nutrition per serving (2 tablespoons): 95 calories; 5g protein; 8g fat (3g sat. fat); 0g carbohydrates; 0g fiber; 0g sugars; 22mg sodium; 7mg calcium; 1mg iron; 80mg potassium; 0mg Vitamin C; 0IU Vitamin A

SMASHES

These are probably the easiest recipes in the entire book. Just peel, and, in the case of the avocado, pit, and mash with a fork. Freeze any leftovers.

BANANA

High in potassium and fiber, creamy bananas are delicious on their own or mixed with cereal or other fruit purées. Choose a nicely ripe banana; it will taste better and be easier to mash.

Nutrition per serving (2 tablespoons): 25 calories; 0g protein; 0g fat (0g sat. fat); 6g carbohydrates; 1g fiber; 3g sugars; 0mg sodium; 1mg calcium; 0mg iron; 100mg potassium; 3mg Vitamin C; 18IU Vitamin A

AVOCADO

With healthy fat and fiber, avocados are wonderful nourishment for your baby. Look for an avocado that gives slightly when you press it. Serve as is, or mixed with yogurt, chicken, or fish.

Nutrition per serving (2 tablespoons): 46 calories; 1g protein; 4g fat (1g sat. fat); 2g carbohydrates; 2g fiber; 0g sugars; 2mg sodium; 4mg calcium; 0mg iron; 139mg potassium; 3mg Vitamin C; 42IU Vitamin A

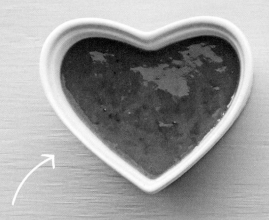

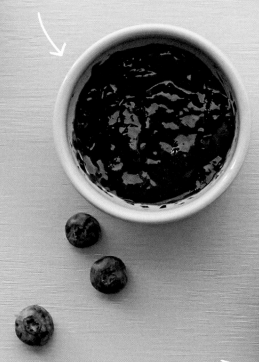

BLUEBERRY PURÉE

Makes about 1½ cups

Purée 1 pint blueberries in a blender.
Strain through a fine-mesh sieve.

STRAWBERRY PURÉE

Makes about ¾ cup

Blend 8 oz. strawberries (about
1½ cups) in a blender.

PEACH PURÉE

Makes about 1 cup

Thaw a 1-pound bag of frozen peaches.
Blend in a food processor or blender
with a little water if needed.

MANGO PURÉE

Makes about ⅓ cup

Blend ¾ cup mango chunks
(about 1 mango peeled and diced)
in a blender.

NO-COOK FRUIT PURÉES

Blending up these brightly colored fruit purées couldn't
be simpler. Serve solo, or mix 2 tablespoons of fruit purée
with ¼ cup plain yogurt for a creamy treat that's just kissed
with sweetness. Start now getting your little one used to
yogurt that isn't overly sugary.

PRUNE PURÉE

Makes about ½ cup

Soak ½ cup pitted prunes in ½ cup hot
water for 20 minutes. Blend the prunes
and the soaking water in a blender.

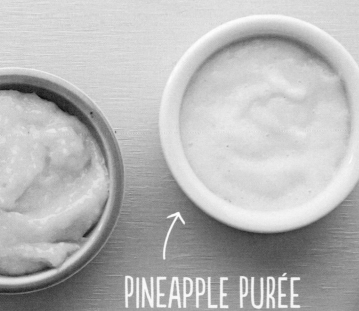

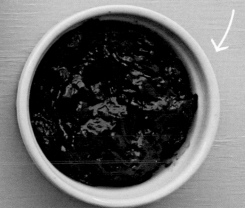

PINEAPPLE PURÉE

Makes about 1½ cups

Blend 2 cups pineapple chunks in
a blender.

SPINACH PURÉE

**ONE 10-OZ. PACKAGE
FROZEN CHOPPED SPINACH**

Unlike some other leafy greens, vitamin A-rich spinach doesn't have a particularly bitter flavor, making it a good "gateway" green.

1 Defrost the spinach according to the package directions. Let cool for at least 10 minutes, reserving any liquid.

2 Transfer the spinach and its liquid to a blender. Process until you get the desired consistency for your baby, adding a tablespoon or more water if needed to help it blend.

Makes about 1⅓ cups

FLAVOR KICK: Purée with a pinch of nutmeg.

Nutrition per serving (2 tablespoons): 8 calories; 1g protein; 0g fat (0g sat. fat); 1g carbohydrates; 1g fiber; 0g sugars; 19mg sodium; 33mg calcium; 1mg iron; 98mg potassium; 1mg Vitamin C; 3027IU Vitamin A

SALMON PURÉE

Sometimes my daughter and I play the, "What are the 10 healthiest foods?" game. (Don't you play this at your house?) My top answer is always salmon, and that goes double for babies whose growing brains crave the DHA found in this incredibly healthy fish.

1 LB. SALMON FILLETS, PREFERABLY WILD, SKINNED

1 In a large saucepan or wide-bottomed pot, bring 2 inches of water to a simmer. Add the salmon fillets in a single layer, making sure they are covered by water. Add more water if necessary. Adjust the heat so the water bubbles gently, cover, and poach until the fish is cooked through, 8 to 10 minutes. Cool slightly, reserving the cooking water.

2 Break the salmon into pieces, and transfer to a blender with ¼ cup of the cooking water. Process until you get the desired consistency for your baby, adding a tablespoon or more water if needed to help it blend.

Makes about 2 cups

FLAVOR KICK: Purée with 1 teaspoon lemon zest.

WHOLESOME TIP

Opt for wild salmon when you can find it, especially when it's fresh and in season during the summer months. Not only is wild salmon usually tastier and more environmentally friendly than farmed salmon, it is lower in saturated fat, higher in iron, and contains a greater proportion of omega-3 relative to total fat. But if you can't find wild salmon or it's too pricey, a sustainably farmed version is undoubtedly better than no salmon at all.

Nutrition per serving (2 tablespoons): 40 calories; 6g protein; 2g fat (0g sat. fat); 2g carbohydrates; 0g fiber; 0g sugars; 32mg sodium; 3mg calcium; 0mg iron; 97mg potassium; 0mg Vitamin C; 54mIU Vitamin A

CHICKEN PURÉE

1 LB. GROUND CHICKEN, PREFERABLY ORGANIC

You could poach a chicken breast and then blend it, but starting with ground chicken makes puréeing much easier.

1 Heat a medium skillet over medium-high heat. Add the chicken and sauté until no longer pink, 5 to 7 minutes. Cool slightly.

2 Transfer the chicken to a blender. Process until you get the desired consistency for your baby, adding a tablespoon or more water if needed to help it blend.

Makes about 1¾ cups

FLAVOR KICK: Purée with ½ teaspoon chopped fresh rosemary.

Turkey Purée: Use ground turkey instead of chicken. Makes about 1 cup.

Nutrition per serving (2 tablespoons): 44 calories; 5g protein; 3g fat (1g sat. fat); 0g carbohydrates; 0g fiber; 0g sugars; 67mg sodium; 2mg calcium; 0mg iron; 161mg potassium; 0mg Vitamin C; 0IU Vitamin A

BLACK BEAN PURÉE *Three Ways*

It couldn't be simpler to blend up canned beans, but cooking beans from scratch is hardly more difficult. Here are three methods for getting this protein rich food ready for your baby.

1 **The Old-Fashioned Way:** Soak 1 pound of dried black beans in a big bowl of water overnight. Drain. Bring a large pot of water to a boil. Add the beans and simmer until tender, 1 to 2 hours. Store the beans in the cooking liquid.

OR

Low and Slow: Rinse 1 pound of dried black beans and add them to a slow cooker. Cover with water by at least 2 inches. Cover the slow cooker and cook on Low for 8 hours or until tender. Store the beans in the cooking liquid.

OR

Instant Gratification: Open a 15-ounce can of low-sodium black beans. Drain and rinse.

2 Transfer the beans to a blender with ¼ cup of water or cooking liquid. Process until you get the desired consistency for your baby, adding a tablespoon or more water if needed to help it blend.

Makes about 1½ cups

FLAVOR KICK: Purée with 2 teaspoons lime juice.

AGE IT UP: Add some salt and finely chopped garlic and you have a delicious spread for tostadas or quesadillas, or a dip for tortilla chips.

1½ CUPS COOKED BLACK BEANS

Nutrition per serving (2 tablespoons): 28 calories; 2g protein; 0g fat (0g sat. fat); 5g carbohydrates; 2g fiber; 0g sugars; 0mg sodium; 6mg calcium; 0mg iron; 76mg potassium; 0mg Vitamin C; 1IU Vitamin A

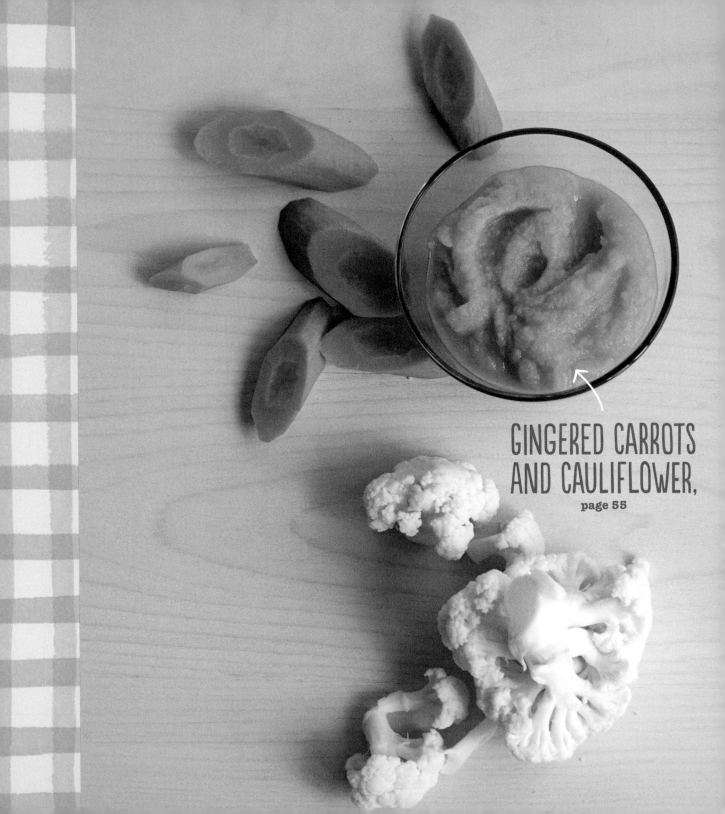

GINGERED CARROTS
AND CAULIFLOWER,
page 55

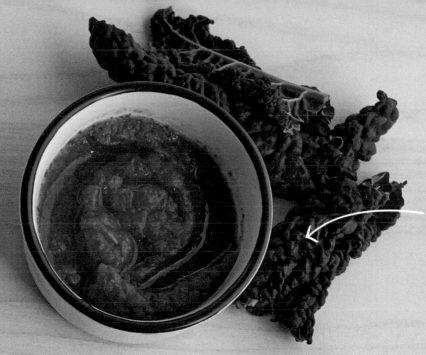

BUTTERNUT SQUASH AND KALE COMBO, page 54

BEGINNING BLENDS

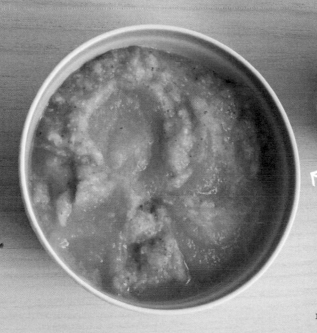

BROCCOLI-APPLE SWIRL

Steam 4 cups broccoli florets until tender, about 10 minutes. Cool slightly and transfer to a blender with ¼ cup water. Blend until desired consistency, adding a bit of water if needed to help it blend. Stir into ¾ cup Apple Purée, page 30. Makes about 2 cups.

BUTTERNUT SQUASH AND KALE COMBO

2½ CUPS CHOPPED KALE,
THICK STEMS REMOVED
(SEE TIP)

2 CUPS BUTTERNUT
SQUASH PURÉE
(SEE PAGE 40)

This blend gives your baby two nutritional power-houses in one spoonful. There are many types of kale available these days. For the quickest cooking time and most tender result, look for Tuscan kale, also called lacinato or dinosaur kale.

1 In a medium saucepan, bring 2 inches of water to a simmer. Place a steamer basket over the water. Add the kale. Cover and steam until tender, about 10 minutes. Cool slightly.

2 Transfer the kale and butternut squash purée to a blender or food processor. Process until you get the desired consistency for your baby, adding ¼ cup or more water if needed to help it blend.

Makes about 2¼ cups

PREPARING STURDY GREENS

To prepare kale or other sturdy greens like Swiss chard and collards, cut out and discard the thick stem in the middle of each leaf. Submerge the leaves in a large bowl of water, swish them around a bit, and let them sit for a couple of minutes. Any dirt clinging to the leaves will sink to the bottom of the bowl. Lift the leaves out of the water and transfer them to a strainer to drain. Pour out the water. Repeat this rinsing process until there's no more dirt at the bottom of the bowl, usually two to three times. Dry the greens in a salad spinner or with towels.

Nutrition per serving (2 tablespoons): 27 calories; 2g protein; 0g fat (0g sat. fat); 7g carbohydrates; 1g fiber; 1g sugars; 6mg sodium; 36mg calcium; 0mg iron; 216mg potassium; 21mg Vitamin C; 6722IU Vitamin A

GINGERED CARROTS AND CAULIFLOWER

Add a hint of spice with ground ginger, or sub in ¼ teaspoon ground cumin for a smokier flavor.

1 In a medium saucepan, bring 2 inches of water to a simmer. Place a steamer basket over the water. Add the carrots. Cover and steam for 5 minutes. Add the cauliflower, cover, and steam until both vegetables are tender, about 10 minutes more. Cool slightly.

2 Transfer the vegetables to a blender or food processor with the ground ginger. Purée until you get the desired consistency for your baby, adding a ¼ cup or more water to the blender if needed to help it blend.

Makes about 2¼ cups

5 CARROTS, PEELED AND CUT INTO ½-INCH THICK COINS

2 CUPS CAULIFLOWER FLORETS

⅛ TEASPOON GROUND GINGER

Nutrition per serving (2 tablespoons): 7 calories; 0g protein; 0g fat (0g sat. fat); 2g carbohydrates; 1g fiber; 2g sugars; 9mg sodium; 5mg calcium; 0mg iron; 45mg potassium; 6mg Vitamin C; 1960IU Vitamin A

RED LENTIL-SPINACH PURÉE ❄

ONE 10-OZ. PACKAGE
FROZEN CHOPPED SPINACH

1½ CUPS RED LENTIL PURÉE
(SEE PAGE 36)

LOW-SODIUM CHICKEN
OR VEGETABLE BROTH,
IF NEEDED

Lentils and spinach combine for a pleasing dish in this smooth and creamy purée.

1 Defrost the spinach according to the package directions. Let cool for at least 10 minutes and drain in a strainer, pressing out the water with a fork.

2 Add the lentil purée and spinach to a blender. Blend until smooth, adding broth by the tablespoon if needed to help it blend.

Makes about 2 cups

Nutrition per serving (2 tablespoons): 16 calories; 2g protein; 0g fat (0g sat. fat); 3g carbohydrates; 1g fiber; 0g sugars; 11mg sodium; 20mg calcium; 1mg iron; 88mg potassium; 1mg Vitamin C; 1665IU Vitamin A

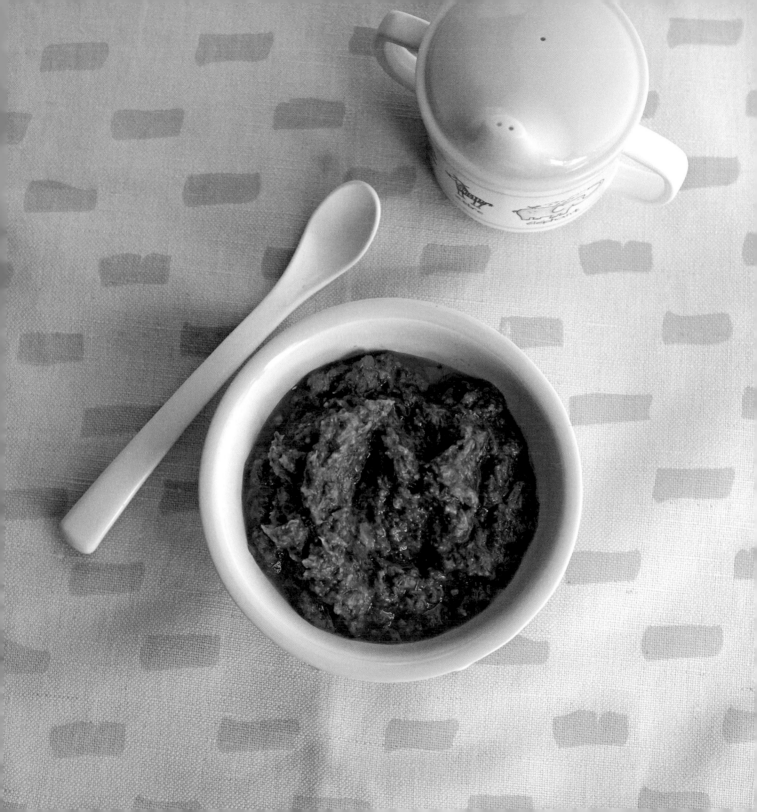

Purée Playdates

Once your baby has tried individual purées, it's time to start making friends. You may find that adding a little apple or potato, say, makes lentils or spinach infinitely more exciting to your little one. There are no hard and fast rules as to what purées blend well, but here are some combinations that are particularly palatable and well-balanced.

	APPLE	POTATO	SWEET POTATO	ZUCCHINI	CAULIFLOWER	B. SQUASH	PEA	LENTIL
APPLE		★	★	★	★	★	★	★
POTATO	★		★	★	★	★	★	★
SWEET POTATO	★	★			★		★	★
ZUCCHINI	★	★			★	★		
CAULIFLOWER	★	★		★		★		
BUTTERNUT SQUASH	★	★		★	★		★	★
PEA	★	★	★		★	★		★
LENTIL	★	★	★	★	★	★	★	
BEEF	★	★	★		★	★	★	★
PEAR	★	★	★	★		★	★	
BROCCOLI	★	★	★	★	★	★		★
SPINACH	★	★	★	★	★	★	★	★
LAMB	★	★	★	★	★	★	★	★
CHICKEN	★	★	★	★	★	★	★	★
TURKEY	★	★	★	★	★	★	★	★
CARROT	★	★		★	★		★	★
PEACH	★	★			★			
BEANS	★	★	★	★	★	★		
SALMON	★	★	★	★	★		★	★

BEEF	PEAR	BROCCOLI	SPINACH	LAMB	CHICKEN	TURKEY	CARROT	PEACH	BEANS	SALMON
★	★	★	★	★	★	★	★	★	★	★
★	★	★	★	★	★	★	★	★	★	★
★	★	★	★	★	★	★			★	★
	★	★	★	★	★	★	★		★	★
★		★	★	★	★	★	★	★		
★	★	★	★	★	★	★			★	
★	★			★	★	★	★			★
★		★	★	★	★	★	★			★
	★	★	★				★	★		
★		★	★	★	★	★	★	★		
★	★			★	★	★	★	★	★	★
★	★			★	★	★	★	★	★	★
	★	★	★				★	★		
	★	★	★				★	★		
	★	★	★				★	★		
★	★	★	★	★	★	★			★	
★	★	★	★	★	★	★			★	★
		★	★				★	★		★
		★	★					★	★	

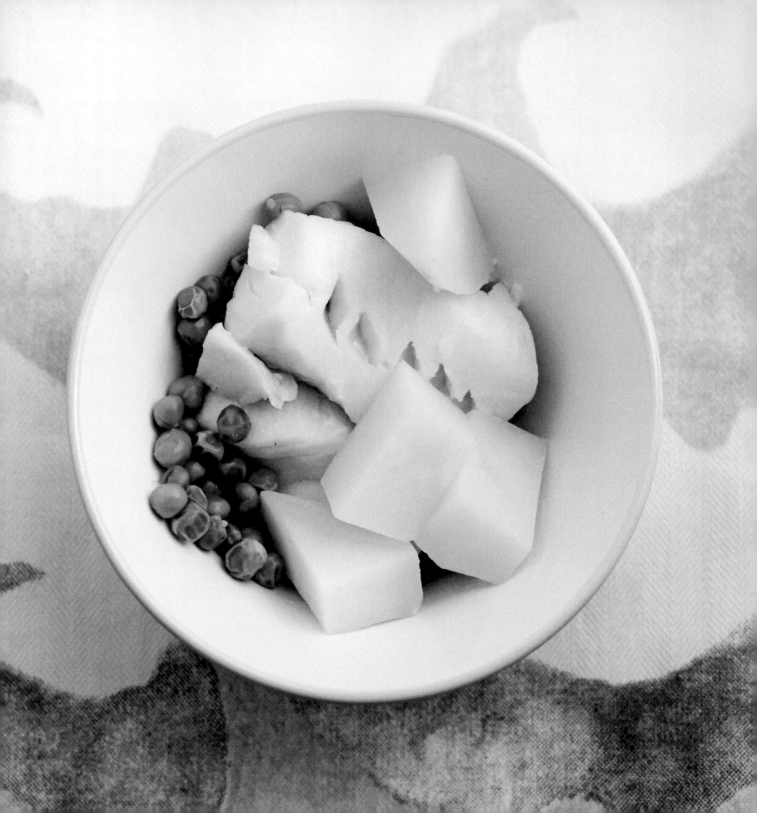

FISH DINNER

Get seafood into your baby's diet early; there are few foods with as many nutritional benefits, including brain-boosting DHA, an especially important omega-3 fatty acid for babies. This mild-tasting, creamy purée is an excellent place to start on the fish front. As your baby gets older, just mash this meal with a fork. Store this purée in the fridge for only a day before freezing to maintain the best (and least "fishy") flavor.

1 MEDIUM YUKON GOLD OR RUSSET POTATO, PEELED AND CUT INTO 1-INCH CUBES

½ POUND COD OR OTHER WHITE FISH FILLET

⅓ CUP FROZEN PEAS

1 Place the potato cubes into a medium saucepan and add water just to cover. Bring to a simmer, cover, and cook for 8 minutes.

2 Place the cod atop the potatoes (it won't be in the water). Cover and cook for 4 minutes. Add the peas and cook for an additional 2 minutes. Cool slightly.

3 Using a slotted spoon, transfer the fish and vegetables to a blender, reserving the cooking water. Add ¼ cup cooking water and purée until the mixture is smooth, adding more cooking water if necessary. Do not over-blend or the potato may become gummy.

Makes about 2½ cups

Nutrition per serving (2 tablespoons): 20 calories; 2g protein; 0g fat (0g sat. fat); 2g carbohydrates; 0g fiber; 0g sugars; 7mg sodium; 4mg calcium; 0mg iron; 97mg potassium; 3mg Vitamin C; 23IU Vitamin A

ZUCCHINI and EGG SCRAMBLE 〔30〕

1 MEDIUM ZUCCHINI, GRATED

1 TEASPOON UNSALTED BUTTER

1 EGG, BEATEN

2 TABLESPOONS BREAST MILK OR FORMULA

Think of this as your baby's first omelet. The zucchini adds a sweet grassy flavor, and the eggs contribute high-quality protein and choline, a mineral essential for eye health.

1 Wrap the grated zucchini in a clean dish towel and squeeze, wringing out as much water as possible.

2 Melt the butter in a small nonstick pan over medium heat. Add the zucchini and cook until soft, about 5 minutes. Add the egg and scramble, stirring until the egg has firmed up. Let cool for a few minutes.

3 Transfer the zucchini-egg mixture to a blender. Add the breast milk or formula and purée until smooth.

Makes about ½ cup

Nutrition per serving (2 tablespoons): 38 calories; 2g protein; 3g fat (1g sat. fat); 2g carbohydrates; 1g fiber; 2g sugars; 21mg sodium; 17mg calcium; 0mg iron; 147mg potassium; 9mg Vitamin C; 205IU Vitamin

Baby-Led Weaning

The basic premise of Baby-Led Weaning (BLW) is that babies do not need any puréed foods in order to successfully transition to solids. In fact, the proponents of this approach claim that feeding babies purées using a spoon may be harmful as it frequently leads to overfeeding and lack of variety in diet.

From about six months of age, babies transitioning to solids using the BLW approach are offered long, graspable pieces of the same foods the family eats. Since the texture is very different from anything they have tried before, babies learn how to chew first, before they learn how to swallow.

Is Baby-Led Weaning better? Babies who are eating family foods are more likely to join families at mealtimes, which has been associated with many positive outcomes in the future. They also get more exposure to wholesome, home-cooked foods. However, parents can achieve these same positive effects by including their baby in family meals and mashing the family's food so the baby can be fed with a spoon.

Proponents of BLW also highlight the method's support of self-regulation in babies and a higher degree of responsiveness demonstrated by parents. But this doesn't mean that spoon-fed babies are automatically disadvantaged. The same benefits can be achieved with spoon-feeding if parents allow their baby to decide how much to eat and stop feeding when he shows signs of fullness.

Will Baby-Led Weaning work for your baby? Choking is the most obvious concern about BLW since babies are expected to suddenly transition from liquid nutrition like milk and formula to very advanced finger foods. But so far limited research has not shown that babies fed the BLW way are at a higher risk.

When considering BLW for your baby, it helps to know that it may work great for some babies and may not work for others. If your child was born prematurely or has oral-motor delays, skipping purées may not be appropriate for him. Besides, not all typically developing babies are able to eat enough finger foods to meet their nutrient needs at six or even eight months. Some nutrients like iron and zinc may be of particular concern since the texture of certain foods like meat may be harder to handle in finger food form.

If you have a family history of food allergies and gluten intolerance, feeding your baby mixed foods from the family table may not be your best bet. If your baby reacts to something in a mixed meal, it will be hard to pinpoint a potential allergen.

If you choose the BLW approach, remain flexible, and be prepared to supplement finger foods with purées, especially if your baby is not able to self-feed by six to seven months.

- Natalia Stasenko, MS, RD

The New Rules for Allergies

Considering waiting until your baby is 12 months or older to introduce fish, nuts, citrus, and eggs? You may not need to. Although traditionally parents have been advised to delay introduction of these and other potentially allergenic foods until babies are one year of age or even older, these recommendations have changed recently as more evidence has mounted that delaying exposure might actually do more harm than good. In 2013 the expert panel from the American Academy of Allergy, Asthma, and Immunology (AAAAI) concluded that there was no evidence to support delaying these foods past the four to six month period when most babies start eating solids. In fact, some preliminary studies show that the later highly allergenic foods are introduced into babies' diets, the more likely a food allergy will develop at some point in their lives.

Foods that are most likely to cause an allergic reaction are:

- Wheat
- Soy
- Nuts
- Eggs
- Fish
- Tree nuts
- Dairy
- Shellfish

According to the AAAAI report, all of these foods can be safely introduced into your baby's diet at around six months of age, as soon as your baby has tried and tolerated a few more traditional solid foods like iron-fortified cereal, fruits, and vegetables.

If you have a strong family history of food allergies or your baby has already been diagnosed with food allergies or severe eczema, talk to your child's doctor before introducing these foods. You will probably need additional instructions as to when and how to introduce them safely.

Some of the foods from the list above may not be good for babies for other reasons. For example, cow's milk is not an appropriate primary drink for babies under 12 months due to its low iron content and low digestibility of protein. However, cheese, yogurt, and the small amount of cow's milk found in baked goods are a safe and nutritious choice for babies less than one year. And although nuts and tree nuts can be a potential choking hazard, nut butter is a perfectly appropriate and nutritious solid food when it is mixed into other purées or thinly spread on toast to be served as a finger food. Feeding nut butters with a spoon is not recommended, however, because they are too thick, sticky, and easy to choke on.

When introducing foods that are more likely to cause an allergic reaction, make sure to start with a very small amount, such as a teaspoon, and do it at home rather than in a daycare or restaurant, preferably in the morning, and observe your baby during the day for signs of allergic reaction. Just as with other solid foods, wait for a couple of days before introducing a new food and increase the amount served gradually.

What does an allergic reaction look like?
Below are potential signs of an allergic reaction. Of course, it will be harder to identify them in nonverbal babies who are not able to explain where it hurts. Your toddler may use a different language to describe what is bothering him, like: "My throat is itchy," "My lips are tight," "It tastes funny," or "It is too spicy."

Mild symptoms of an allergic reaction:

- Hives (reddish, swollen, itchy areas on the skin)
- Eczema (a persistent dry, itchy rash)
- Redness of the skin or around the eyes
- Itchy mouth or ear canal
- Nausea or vomiting
- Diarrhea
- Stomach pain
- Nasal congestion or runny nose
- Sneezing
- Slight, dry cough
- Odd taste in mouth

Severe symptoms of an allergic reaction:

- Obstructive swelling of the lips, tongue, and/or throat
- Trouble swallowing
- Shortness of breath or wheezing
- Turning blue
- Drop in blood pressure (feeling faint, confused, weak, passing out)
- Loss of consciousness
- Chest pain
- A weak or "thread" pulse

If your child develops a severe allergic reaction to a food, typically manifested by a swelling of the face, tongue, and lips, difficulty breathing, coughing, or wheezing, call 911 immediately or get to the closest emergency room. Make sure to discuss milder reactions such as a skin rash or diarrhea with your pediatrician, who may recommend further allergy testing with a specialist. If your child tests positive for a food allergy, it is hard to predict the severity of reaction the next time he eats the food, so your doctor may recommend avoiding it completely.

- Natalia Stasenko, MS, RD

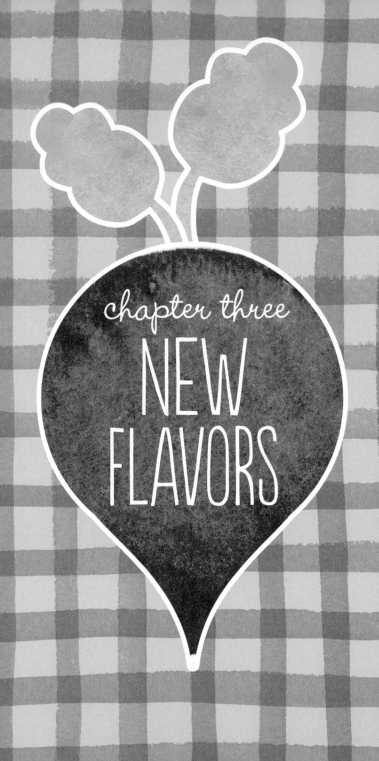

chapter three

NEW FLAVORS

VARIED TASTES FOR OLDER BABIES
(8-12 months)

By now your baby has probably mastered purées and tried a wide variety of nutritious—and delicious—new tastes. It's time to get more adventurous with his meals by introducing fresh flavors and more complex dishes. This is one of my favorite stages in a baby's eating career. By nine months Rosa was more comfortable in the high chair, more at ease with utensils, and just more expressive (dare I say even more cute?). Each day was different, and I was curious to see what flavors she would prefer and whether most of the finger foods would end up in her mouth or on the floor (um, often the floor...this is also when we invested in a small handheld vacuum).

I prepared most of the dishes in this chapter specifically for Rosa, continuing to use the freezer for easy meals during the week. But a few of the recipes (I'm thinking of Baby's Bolognese, Greek Fish and Tomatoes, and Curried Cauliflower and Chickpeas) were our dinnertime standbys that just happened to make delicious, age-appropriate baby food. And sometimes it works the other way around: After making the Rosemary Roasted Pears just for Rosa, I promptly ate half of it myself.

at this stage

Since your baby's tummy is still so tiny, you want to be sure to feed her the most nutrient-dense foods possible, full of protein, iron, and all the vitamins and minerals she needs to be healthy and strong. The recipes in this chapter fit the bill perfectly, chock-full of both nutrition and flavor.

As your baby grows and becomes more proficient at chewing and swallowing, you'll want to maintain more texture in her food. Instead of using a blender, transition to pulsing dishes in a food processor, blending them with a handheld immersion blender, or simply employing a knife and fork to do the job (less dishes!). Don't be afraid to feed your child chunkier foods once she has mastered purées. According to a 2009 study, children who started lumpier foods between six and nine months had more food acceptance at age seven.

During this period you should also offer your baby a wider variety of finger foods. Look for ideas in chapter four.

Continue with a sippy cup of water at each meal. At around eight to ten months it's time to move on to a cup with a straw, which will allow your baby to train another set of muscles and learn new drinking skills. Consider both sippy and straw cups as transitional tools, rather than permanent ways of drinking. By 12 months, your toddler is ready for an open cup. Start experimenting with very small amounts of milk or water and have plenty of kitchen towels at hand during the learning period. This upgrade is extremely important for your child's oral health and development of feeding skills, so don't let the mess deter you (as tempting as that may be).

SERVING SIZES

Your baby will likely be able to handle ¼ cup or more of each of the meals in this chapter. Most of the recipes make many times more than that, so there will be plenty to refrigerate or freeze for future meals.

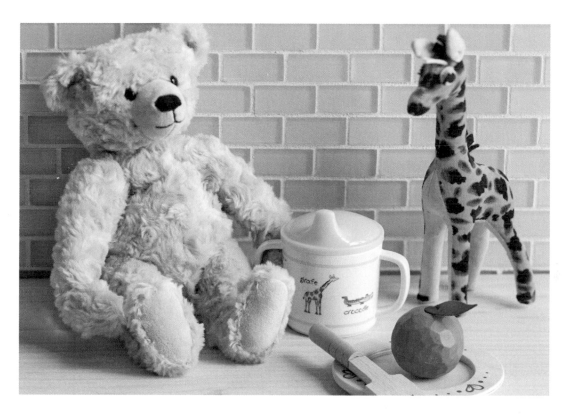

wholesome feeding tips

- Make sure your baby has transitioned to a regular feeding schedule by now, a structure that includes three set meals a day, plus a midmorning and midafternoon snack. Some babies also need a bedtime snack, so be guided by your little one.

- Continue to avoid added salt until your baby is 12 months old, and take this opportunity to attune her palate to foods without a lot of added sugars.

- Babies at this stage love to explore. Let your little one touch and squeeze the food. By ten months he may be ready to practice with a fork and spoon.

- Don't be alarmed if your baby chows down at one meal and then hardly eats at the next, or if he rejects a food he liked just yesterday. Babies' appetites are always in flux, and they are still experimenting with flavors. Trust your baby, and never pressure him to eat.

- Your child may make a funny face when he tries a new food, but don't give up as long as he continues to eat! At this stage most children are open to new foods, so continue to serve a variety and meet your baby's frowns with smiles.

ROSEMARY ROASTED PEARS

4 RIPE (BUT NOT SQUISHY) BARTLETT PEARS (ABOUT 2 LBS)

2 TEASPOONS OLIVE OIL

½ TEASPOON FINELY CHOPPED FRESH ROSEMARY

2 TABLESPOONS ALMOND BUTTER

Give your baby a head start on sophisticated flavors with this delicious twist on basic applesauce.

1 Preheat the oven to 375°F. Line a rimmed baking sheet with parchment paper.

2 Peel and core the pears; slice each into 8 wedges. Toss the pears with the olive oil. Spread them out on the baking sheet and roast for 30 minutes or until tender and lightly golden brown. Cool slightly.

3 Transfer the pears to a medium bowl. Mash the pears with a fork until you get the desired consistency for your baby. Stir in the rosemary and almond butter.

Makes about 2 cups

AGE IT UP: This pear sauce is scrumptious at any age. Make it part of a cheese plate, or spread it between two slices of toast for a satisfying breakfast or lunch.

WHOLESOME TIP
Look for creamy unsweetened and unsalted almond butter.

Nutrition per serving (¼ cup): 100 calories; 1g protein; 4g fat (0g sat. fat); 18g carbohydrates; 4g fiber; 11g sugars; 1mg sodium; 24mg calcium; 0mg iron; 165mg potassium; 5mg Vitamin C; 26IU Vitamin A

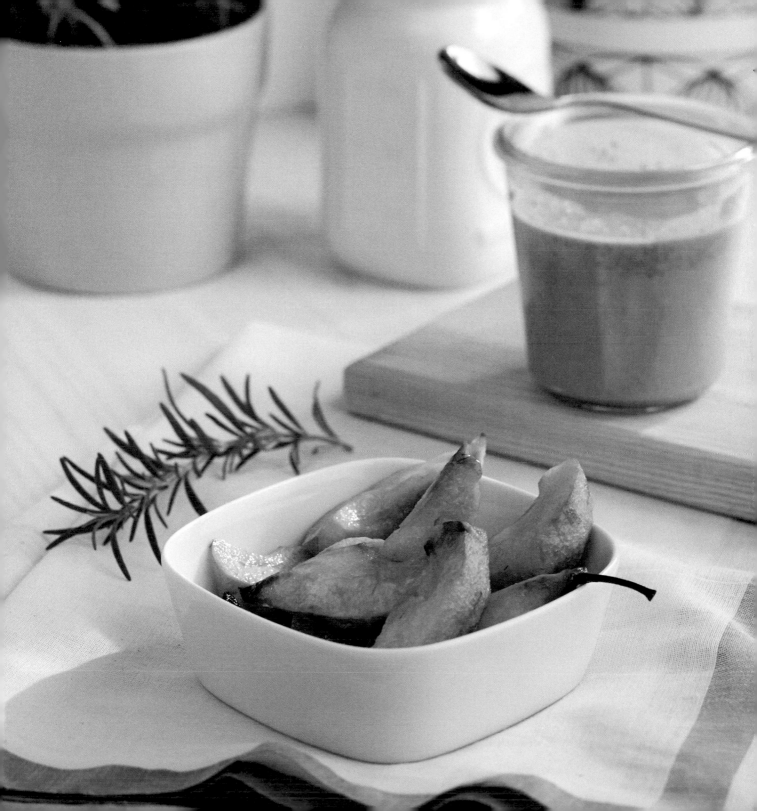

SALMON, KALE, AND SWEET POTATO SMASH

1 MEDIUM SWEET POTATO, PEELED AND CUT INTO 1-INCH CHUNKS

2½ CUPS CHOPPED TUSCAN KALE, THICK STEMS REMOVED

6 OZ. SALMON FILLET, SKINNED AND CUT INTO 4 PIECES

Superfood alert! Salmon, kale, and sweet potatoes all top the list of nutrient and antioxidant-rich foods. Be sure to run your fingers along the salmon to check for small bones. Use regular tweezers or fish tweezers to easily remove them.

1 In a medium saucepan, bring 2 inches of water to a simmer. Place a steamer basket over the water. Add the sweet potato chunks. Cover and steam for 5 minutes.

2 Add the kale and cook for another 3 minutes. Add the salmon and cook for 5 more minutes or until the vegetables are tender and the salmon is cooked through. Cool slightly.

3 Transfer the vegetables and salmon to a bowl. Using an immersion blender, a potato masher, or a fork, mash until you get the desired consistency for your baby.

Makes about 2½ cups

Nutrition per serving (¼ cup): 87 calories; 8g protein; 2g fat (0g sat. fat); 8g carbohydrates; 1g fiber; 1g sugars; 43mg sodium; 57mg calcium; 1mg iron; 404mg potassium; 41mg Vitamin C; 8853IU Vitamin A

SAVORY BEEF AND BROCCOLI

Give your little one a sneak preview of stir-fries to come with this tasty, protein-rich meal.

1 In a medium saucepan, bring the beef broth to a boil. Add the steak, making sure it is covered by the broth (add a bit more if necessary). Place the florets on top of the steak. They don't need to be submerged. Cover the pan, reduce the heat to medium-low, and simmer for 15 minutes or until the steak is cooked through and the broccoli is very tender. Cool slightly.

2 With an immersion blender, food processor, or knife and fork, mash the beef and broccoli until you get the desired consistency for your baby.

Makes about 2 cups

¾ CUP LOW-SODIUM BEEF BROTH

½ LB. STRIP STEAK OR TOP SIRLOIN, FAT TRIMMED AND CUT INTO CUBES

3 CUPS BROCCOLI FLORETS

Nutrition per serving (¼ cup): 88 calories; 15g protein; 2g fat (1g sat. fat); 4g carbohydrates; 2g fiber; 1g sugars; 97mg sodium; 28mg calcium; 1mg iron; 365mg potassium; 38mg Vitamin C; 905IU Vitamin A

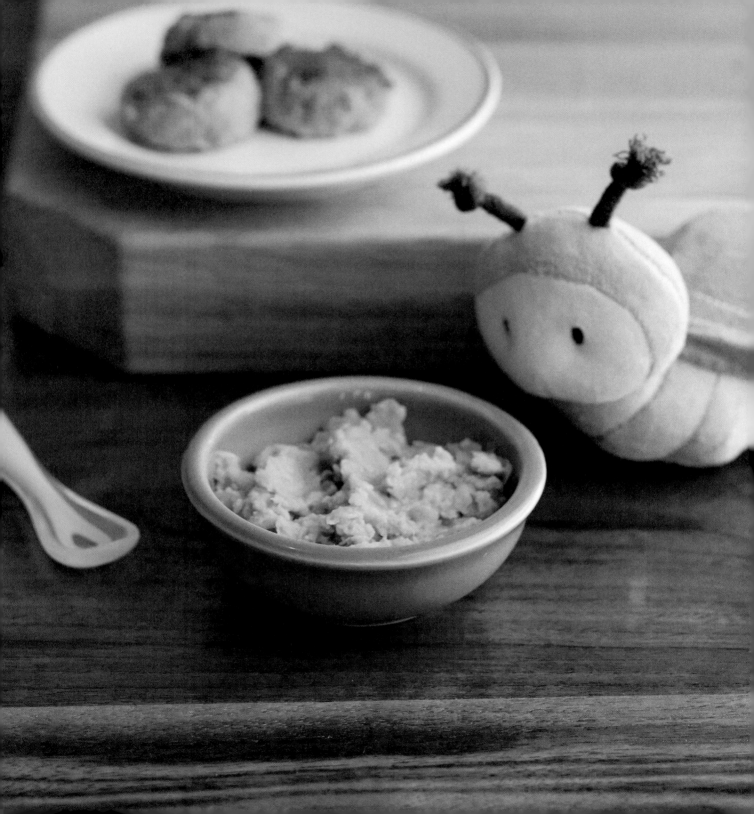

CURRIED CAULIFLOWER AND CHICKPEAS

Cauliflower, chickpeas, and curry are a classic Indian flavor combination.

1 In a medium saucepan, bring the chicken broth and water to a boil. Add the cauliflower florets and the chickpeas. They won't be covered by the liquid. Cover the pan, reduce the heat to medium-low, and simmer for 8 to 10 minutes or until the cauliflower is very tender. Cool slightly.

2 Sprinkle in the curry powder. With an immersion blender, food processor, or knife and fork, mash the cauliflower and chickpeas until you get the desired consistency for your baby.

Makes about 3 cups

AGE IT UP: For a delicious snack or lunch for kids and grown-ups of all ages, add a beaten egg, ½ teaspoon salt, extra curry powder to taste, and enough panko for the veggies to come together. Form into cakes and sauté in olive oil until golden brown.

½ CUP LOW-SODIUM CHICKEN BROTH (OR VEGETABLE BROTH OR WATER)

½ CUP WATER

4 CUPS CAULIFLOWER FLORETS (ABOUT HALF A HEAD)

1 CUP CANNED CHICKPEAS, RINSED AND DRAINED

½ TEASPOON MILD CURRY POWDER

Nutrition per serving (¼ cup): 63 calories; 3g protein; 1g fat (0g sat. fat); 12g carbohydrates; 3g fiber; 1g sugars; 140mg sodium; 24mg calcium; 0mg iron; 232mg potassium; 25mg Vitamin C; 8IU Vitamin A

COMFORTING CHICKEN SOUP

1½ TEASPOONS UNSALTED BUTTER

1 LEEK, WHITE AND LIGHT GREEN PARTS ONLY, CHOPPED

½ CUP LOW-SODIUM CHICKEN BROTH

½ CUP WATER

1 MEDIUM YUKON GOLD POTATO, PEELED AND CHOPPED

2 CARROTS, PEELED AND CHOPPED

1 BONELESS, SKINLESS CHICKEN BREAST, CUT INTO 1-INCH CHUNKS

1 TEASPOON LEMON JUICE

Let your baby find out early how satisfying chicken soup can be.

1 Melt the butter in a medium saucepan over medium-low heat. Add the leek and cook until tender, about 5 minutes.

2 Add the chicken broth, water, potatoes, and carrots to the pan. Bring to a boil. Reduce the heat to low, cover, and simmer for 10 minutes. Add the chicken, cover, and simmer for 8 more minutes or until the chicken is cooked through and the vegetables are tender. Cool slightly.

3 Add the lemon juice. With an immersion blender, food processor, or knife and fork, mash the chicken and veggies until you get the desired consistency for your baby.

Makes about 2¾ cups

WHOLESOME TIP

When buying canned goods, always look for cans that haven't been lined with BPA, a chemical that may have negative effects on developing brains. Or, seek out boxed or pouched versions.

Nutrition per serving (¼ cup): 115 calories; 5g protein; 3g fat (1g sat. fat); 18g carbohydrates; 2g fiber; 1g sugars; 44mg sodium; 26mg calcium; 1mg iron; 346mg potassium; 13mg Vitamin C; 2145IU Vitamin A

BABY'S BOLOGNESE

This recipe will keep you in sauce for the foreseeable future, and you'll be glad once you see how much your little one loves it. Freeze some in small quantities to defrost quickly for your baby's meals; freeze the rest in larger portions for the whole family to eat over pasta.

1 Heat the olive oil in a medium-sized pot. Add the ground beef, onion, carrots, and garlic. Sauté over medium heat until the beef is no longer pink, about 8 to 10 minutes. Drain and return to the pot.

2 Add the rosemary and stir to combine. Add the chicken broth and tomatoes. Bring the sauce to a boil. Reduce the heat to a simmer and cook, stirring occasionally, for 30 minutes. Remove from the heat and stir in the ricotta cheese.

3 To serve, mix ¼ cup cooked orzo with 2 tablespoons of sauce. With an immersion blender, food processor, or knife and fork, mash the pasta and sauce until you get the desired consistency for your baby.

Makes about 5 cups sauce

AGE IT UP: Add 1¼ teaspoons salt and a pinch of sugar to the sauce.

1 TABLESPOON OLIVE OIL

1 LB. GROUND BEEF

1 CUP FINELY CHOPPED ONION

2 MEDIUM CARROTS, PEELED AND FINELY CHOPPED

1 CLOVE GARLIC, FINELY CHOPPED

½ TEASPOON CHOPPED FRESH ROSEMARY

1 CUP LOW-SODIUM CHICKEN BROTH

ONE 28-OZ. CAN CRUSHED TOMATOES

2 TABLESPOONS RICOTTA CHEESE

For serving:

¼ CUP COOKED WHOLE-WHEAT ORZO

Nutrition per serving: 30 calories; 3g protein; 1g fat (0g sat. fat); 2g carbohydrates; 1g fiber; 1g sugars; 51mg sodium; 12mg calcium; 1mg iron; 115mg potassium; 2mg Vitamin C; 538IU Vitamin A

Sweet Spiced
CHICKEN STEW

⅓ CUP LOW-SODIUM CHICKEN BROTH

½ CUP WATER

1 BONELESS, SKINLESS CHICKEN BREAST, CUT INTO 2-INCH CHUNKS

1 MEDIUM ZUCCHINI, THINLY SLICED INTO HALF MOONS

4 PITTED PRUNES, CHOPPED

½ TEASPOON CINNAMON

½ TEASPOON GROUND CUMIN

An immersion blender works particularly well when mashing this lightly spiced stew. Don't be tempted to leave out the prunes. They add a deep and pleasing sweetness, plus they are excellent for your baby's digestive health.

1 In a medium saucepan, bring the chicken broth and water to a boil. Add the chicken. Cover the pan, reduce the heat to medium-low, and simmer for 5 minutes.

2 Add the zucchini, prunes, cinnamon, and cumin and stir. Cover and simmer for 10 minutes or until the chicken is cooked through and the zucchini is tender. Uncover and cool slightly.

3 With an immersion blender, food processor, or knife and fork, mash the stew until you get the desired consistency for your baby.

Makes about 2 cups

Nutrition per serving (¼ cup): 53 calories; 8g protein; 1g fat (0g sat. fat); 4g carbohydrates; 1g fiber; 2g sugars; 20mg sodium; 10mg calcium; 0mg iron; 152mg potassium; 4mg Vitamin C; 90IU Vitamin A

MIGHTY GREEN BEANS

Quinoa and almond butter add a punch of protein to this appealing dish.

1 Preheat the oven to 425°F. Line a rimmed baking sheet with parchment paper.

2 Toss the green beans with the olive oil. Spread on the prepared baking sheet and roast until tender, 15 to 20 minutes.

3 In a large bowl, combine the green beans with the quinoa, almond butter, and mint leaves. Add 2 tablespoons of water. With an immersion blender, food processor, or knife and fork, mash the stew until you get the desired consistency for your baby. Add a tablespoon or more water if needed for smoother blending.

Makes about 2 cups

1 LB. GREEN BEANS, TRIMMED

2 TEASPOONS OLIVE OIL

1½ CUPS COOKED QUINOA

2 TABLESPOONS ALMOND BUTTER

4 MINT LEAVES, CHOPPED

Nutrition per serving (¼ cup): 98 calories; 4g protein; 4g fat (0g sat. fat); 12g carbohydrates; 3g fiber; 2g sugars; 4mg sodium; 51mg calcium; 1mg iron; 272mg potassium; 5mg Vitamin C; 2IU Vitamin A

BEETS IN YOGURT WITH DILL

1½ CUPS CHOPPED, COOKED BEETS (ABOUT 10 OZ.)

2 TABLESPOONS PLAIN, WHOLE-MILK GREEK YOGURT

⅛ TEASPOON CHOPPED DILL

Forget the fact that these beets are smooth, creamy, and surprisingly sweet. They are worth making for the bright magenta color alone.

1 Purée the beets in a blender until smooth.

2 To serve, stir together 2 tablespoons beet purée with the 2 tablespoons Greek yogurt. Sprinkle with the dill.

Makes about 1½ cups

Nutrition per serving (¼ cup): 40 calories; 3g protein; 2g fat (1g sat. fat); 4g carbohydrates; 1g fiber; 3g sugars; 37mg sodium; 44mg calcium; 0mg iron; 87mg potassium; 5mg Vitamin C; 438IU Vitamin A

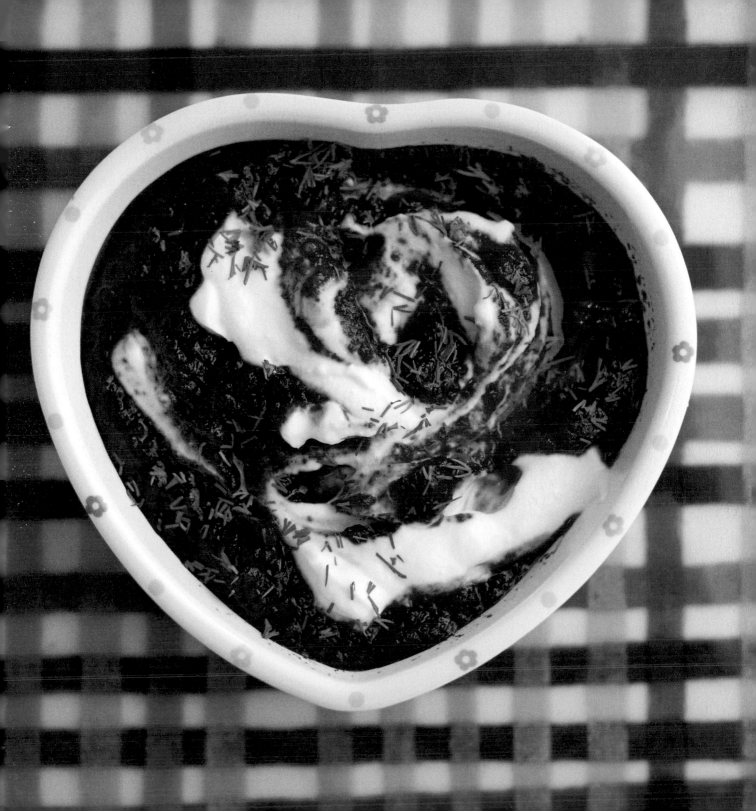

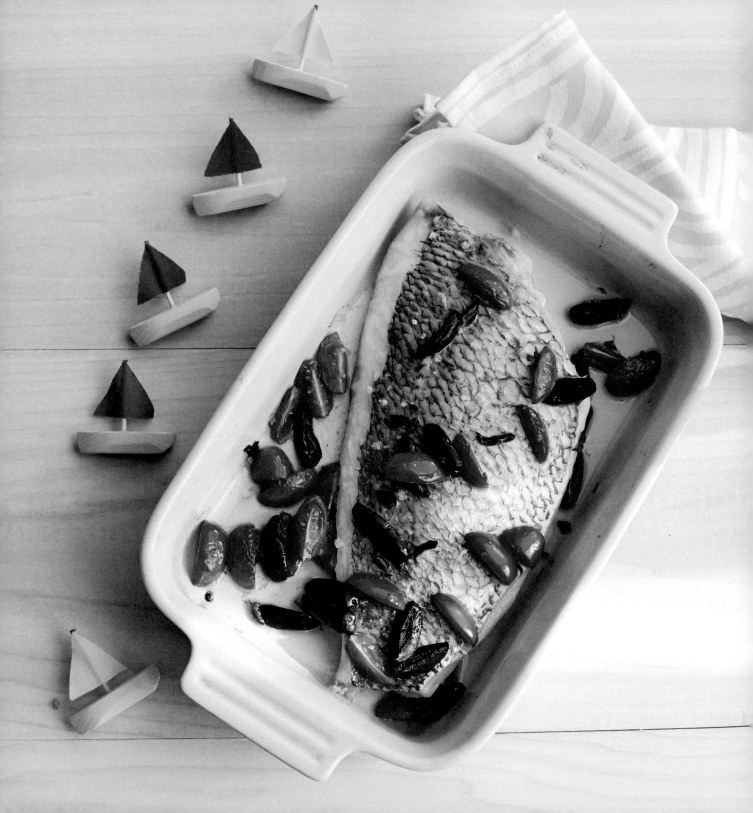

GREEK FISH and TOMATOES

I make a variation of this dish for my (grown-up!) personal chef clients. For a hit of brine I always roast some capers or pitted Kalamata olives along with the tomatoes. Let your older baby explore these flavors as well by serving them on the side.

1 Preheat the oven to 400°F. Rub a small baking pan with olive oil.

2 Place the snapper on the prepared pan. Drizzle with ¼ teaspoon olive oil, spreading it over the fish with the back of a spoon or your fingers.

3 In a small bowl, combine the tomatoes, olives or capers, ½ teaspoon olive oil, and oregano. Spoon over the fish. Most of it will land on the pan; that's fine. Roast until the fish flakes easily with a fork, about 10 minutes. Cool slightly.

4 Transfer the fish, tomatoes and any juices to a large bowl, leaving behind the olives or capers and the fish's skin. With an immersion blender, food processor, or knife and fork, mash the fish and tomatoes until you get the desired consistency for your baby. Serve the olives or capers on the side.

Makes about 1 cup

AGE IT UP: Before mashing, this is a lovely, easy dinner for the grown-ups and big kids in the household. Just salt and pepper the grown-up's portions.

OLIVE OIL

6 OZ. RED SNAPPER FILLET OR OTHER WHITE FISH, BONES REMOVED

½ CUP GRAPE TOMATOES, QUARTERED

2 TABLESPOONS PITTED KALAMATA OLIVES, HALVED, OR 2 TEASPOONS CAPERS

¼ TEASPOON DRIED OREGANO

Nutrition per serving (¼ cup): 53 calories; 8g protein; 1.8g fat (0g sat. fat); 1g carbohydrates; 0g fiber; 1g sugars; 55mg sodium; 9mg calcium; 0mg iron; 229mg potassium; 4mg Vitamin C; 204IU Vitamin A

PUMPKIN-BANANA MASH

1 TEASPOON UNSALTED
BUTTER

1 MEDIUM BANANA, SLICED

¼ CUP CANNED
PUMPKIN PURÉE

⅛ TEASPOON CINNAMON

What a treat! Buttery-soft banana is mixed with smooth and creamy pumpkin purée and spiked with cinnamon. Be sure to use a ripe banana for the sweetest flavor.

1 Melt the butter in a medium skillet over medium heat. Add the banana slices and sauté until lightly browned, about 5 minutes.

2 Transfer the banana to a small bowl. Add the pumpkin and cinnamon. With a fork, mash the banana to get the desired consistency for your baby.

Makes about ½ cup

Nutrition per serving (¼ cup): 95 calories; 1g protein; 2g fat (1g sat. fat); 20g carbohydrates; 3g fiber; 10g sugars; 3mg sodium; 14mg calcium; 1mg iron; 332mg potassium; 8mg Vitamin C; 4877IU Vitamin A

FRUITY TOFU PUDDING

Make this creamy concoction a day ahead, and feel free to experiment with different fruits.

1. Put all of the ingredients in a food processor and process until smooth, stopping occasionally to scrape down the sides with a rubber spatula.

2. Transfer the pudding to a storage container and refrigerate for at least 4 hours or overnight.

Makes about 1 cup

Nutrition per serving (¼ cup): 66 calories; 3g protein; 2g fat (0g sat. fat); 10g carbohydrates; 1g fiber; 8g sugars; 3mg sodium; 21mg calcium; 1mg iron; 185mg potassium; 4mg Vitamin C; 121IU Vitamin A

8 OZ. SILKEN TOFU, LIQUID POURED OFF

1 CUP CHOPPED NECTARINE (ABOUT 1)

¼ CUP RASPBERRIES

1 TABLESPOON AGAVE NECTAR

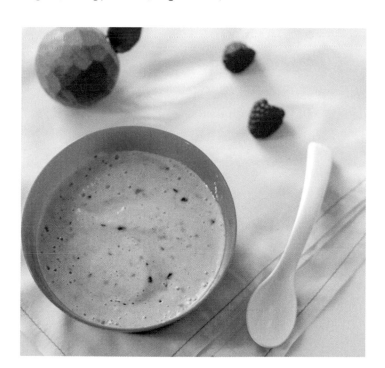

WHOLESOME TIP

Tofu is a wonderful addition to the diet of vegetarian and non-vegetarian babies alike. Inexpensive and high in protein, it has a mild flavor that plays well with both sweet and savory ingredients.

Raising a Vegetarian or Vegan Baby and Toddler

A well-planned vegetarian or vegan diet is not only totally appropriate for a baby and a toddler, it may be even more nutritious than a standard American diet. However, it is also very easy to fall short on certain nutrients, so parents need to take extra care to be sure their children are receiving all of the vitamins and minerals they need to grow into strong, healthy tots.

IMPORTANT NUTRIENTS FOR VEGETARIAN OR VEGAN BABIES

Iron and zinc are key nutrients for all babies to consume during the introduction of solids, but it can be especially challenging for vegetarian and vegan babies to get enough, especially if they are breastfed.

If you are breastfeeding your vegetarian or vegan baby, be sure that good sources of iron and zinc are introduced into his diet when you first start solids. Aim to provide 11 grams of iron and three grams of zinc per day for a baby under 12 months. Iron-fortified cereals, nut butters, tofu, beans, and eggs are all rich sources of iron and zinc. And don't forget about leafy green vegetables steamed, puréed, and mixed with avocado, applesauce, cottage cheese, and yogurt, or purées such as apple, potato, sweet potato, zucchini, and cauliflower (see recipes in chapter two).

Since formula provides all of the iron and zinc babies need in the first year, formula-fed babies are more likely to meet their requirements. But it still very helpful to introduce iron and zinc-rich foods so that by the time children switch to dairy or non-dairy milks at 12 months of age, toddlers have well-established sources of these crucial minerals in their diets.

Be aware that some vegetarian sources of zinc are also high in phytates, a chemical compound that inhibits zinc absorption. Phytates are found in nuts, whole grains, and soy products. While cooking somewhat reduces phytate levels, overnight soaking, fermentation, and sprouting are even more effective. Some experts suggest increasing intake of zinc and iron by up to 50 percent for strict vegans, but the exact way to calculate the amount of absorbed nutrients is not known. Make sure to discuss a supplement with your doctor or dietitian if you think your baby is not getting enough iron or zinc.

IMPORTANT NUTRIENTS FOR VEGETARIAN OR VEGAN TODDLERS

After 12 months, full-fat cow's milk provides healthy fats, protein, and calcium for omnivore and vegetarian babies. If your baby is vegan, fortified soy milk with calcium, vitamin B12, and vitamin D will be the best substitute for cow's milk since it has a similar nutritional content. Other plant milks like hemp milk, rice milk, and almond milk are too low in protein and/or fat to be a primary drink for

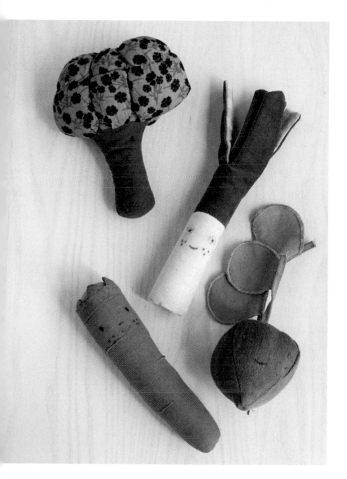

toddlers under two years of age, although it is okay to serve them occasionally.

Iron and zinc continue to be important, although toddlers need a little less iron—7mg a day instead of 11mg for infants.

Omega-3 fatty acids are crucial for brain development in the first two years of life. Cold-water fish is the best source of these fats. In order to be used by our bodies as DHA (a form of omega-3 that is especially beneficial for babies and toddlers) and EPA (another form of omega-3), plant forms of omega-3 (ALA) need to undergo an additional conversion, which makes them less bio-available, and a supplement may be necessary for vegan children under two. For older children, ground flax seeds, flaxseed oil, chia seeds, walnuts, and canola oil are all good sources of omega-3 if fish is not on the menu.

Vitamin D can become a concern for a vegan baby and toddler because it is found in its natural form only in animal products. Many dairy products like milk and yogurt, as well as vegan soy-based formulas, are fortified with vitamin D, as are many brands of soy milk and orange juice. Sun exposure two to three times weekly for 20 to 30 minutes without wearing a sunscreen may be a reliable way to get enough vitamin D. If your vegan child is not getting enough sun exposure, take extra care to buy fortified beverages or consider vitamin D supplements. Babies under 12 months need 400IU of vitamin D and toddlers need 600IU.

MEATLESS SOURCES OF KEY NUTRIENTS FOR BABIES AND TODDLERS

IRON	ZINC	OMEGA-3	VITAMIN D	VITAMIN B12
11mg for babies and 7mg for toddlers	3mg for babies from 7 months and toddlers	DHA: 100-150 mg per day OR ALA: 0.3-0.5g per day	400IU for babies and 600IU for toddlers	0.5mcg for babies and 0.9mcg for toddlers
Breakfast cereals, fortified with 100% of the DV for iron, 1 serving (check the label for serving size) - 18mg	Breakfast cereal, fortified with 25% of the DV for zinc, ¾ cup serving - 3.8mg	Salmon, wild, cooked, 1 oz. - 235 mg DHA	Salmon, wild, cooked, 1 oz. - 149IU	Breakfast cereals fortified with 100% DV, 1 serving - 6 mcg
Lentils, boiled and drained, ½ cup - 3mg	Tofu, raw, regular, ¼ cup - 0.5 mg	Sardines, canned in oil, drained, 1 oz. - 144 mg DHA	Tuna fish, canned in water, drained, 1 oz. - 51IU	Trout, rainbow, wild, cooked, 1 oz. - 1.8 mcg
Tofu, raw, regular, ¼ cup - 3.3 mg	Chickpeas, cooked, ½ cup - 1.3mg	Walnuts, shelled, 1 oz. - 2.6 g ALA	Orange juice fortified with vitamin D, 1 cup - 137IU	Salmon, sockeye, cooked, 1 oz. - 1.5 mcg
Kidney beans, canned, ½ cup - 2mg	Peanut butter, 1 tbsp. - 0.45mg	Kale, cooked, ½ cup - 67mg ALA	Milk, vitamin D-fortified, 1 cup - 115-124IU	Egg - 0.6mcg
Raisins, seedless, ¼ cup - 1mg	Peas, green, frozen, cooked, ½ cup - 0.5mg	Flaxseeds, ground, 1 tsp. - 570 mg ALA	Egg, 1 large (vitamin D is found in yolk) - 41IU	Milk, 1 cup - 1.2 mcg
Egg, 1 large - 0.8 mg	Egg, 1 large - 0.6 mg	Chia seeds, 1 oz. - 5g ALA	Soy milk, fortified with vitamin D, 1 cup - 100IU	Hard cheese 1 oz. - 0.9mcg

Finally, vitamin B12 is only found in animal products. Formula is fortified with vitamin B12; levels of vitamin B12 in breast milk depend on the mother's diet. As babies start eating more solids their intake of both formula and breast milk goes down and getting enough vitamin B12 through solids becomes important. If your baby is vegan, make sure to discuss a supplement with your doctor or include a variety of vitamin B12-fortified products in her diet, such as nutritional yeast, cereals, milk alternatives, and meat analogues.

Keep in mind that vegetarian, and especially vegan, diets may be very bulky because of high fiber intake from whole grains, beans, and lentils. Since toddlers have little stomachs, they may feel full before meeting their caloric and nutrient needs, and this may result in too-slow weight gain. To ease up on the fiber, try mixing whole grains with refined grains and peel fruit and vegetables occasionally. Remember to always serve a good source of fat at each meal, such as plant oils, avocados, and nut butters, to add calories and nutrition to the diet.

Your best strategy may be to consult your doctor or a registered dietitian to get a personalized assessment and action plan to make sure your baby and toddler are getting all the nutrition they need in this period of fast growth and development.

- Natalia Stasenko, MS, RD

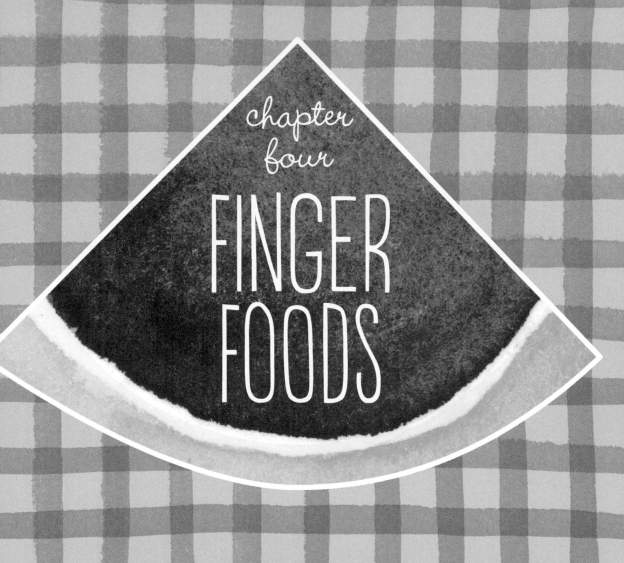

chapter
four

FINGER
FOODS

FUN BITES FOR GROWING EATERS
(8 months and up)

Many a parent has mastered purées only to be thrown a curve ball when the finger food stage rolls around. "What's a good finger food?" more than one of my mom friends has asked me. Giving your tiny baby truly solid food seems risky; there must be lots of do's and don'ts about what to feed, right?

The truth is, as long as a food is soft enough and small enough, it probably makes a good finger food. My niece loves torn up pancakes and shredded cheese. My nephew adored fruit, fruit, and more fruit. My daughter ate up anything savory, such as meatloaf or eggs. The key to finger foods is to just go for it. Make one of the easy recipes in this chapter or even cut up some of your own food into small pieces. The most important rule: don't stress. Finger foods are just one more milestone on the road to eating independence.

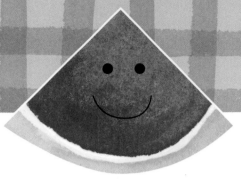

at this stage

Finger foods are a crucial part of your baby's transition to solids. In addition to helping your little one become a more grown-up eater, picking up small bits of food will promote hand-eye coordination.

Start offering small amounts of finger foods when your baby first begins eating solids. Smart early options include tried-and-true Cheerios, small pieces of fruit, and very soft, chopped, cooked vegetables. Once your baby has gotten the hang of feeding herself, either by picking food up with her palm, or later, with her fingers, quickly start making finger foods a larger part of your baby's meals with more interesting options, like the recipes in this chapter. At first, it may seem like your baby is doing more gnawing than actually chewing and swallowing. This is normal; at about eight to ten months old her self-feeding will become much more coordinated, and finger foods can help add important nutrients to her diet.

Be aware that babies with an independent streak may prefer finger foods to purées altogether, and if you're following the Baby-Led Weaning method (see page 63) of transitioning your baby to grown-up food, the recipes in this chapter could become your best friends. But most babies will enjoy finger foods in conjunction with the other meals you're serving.

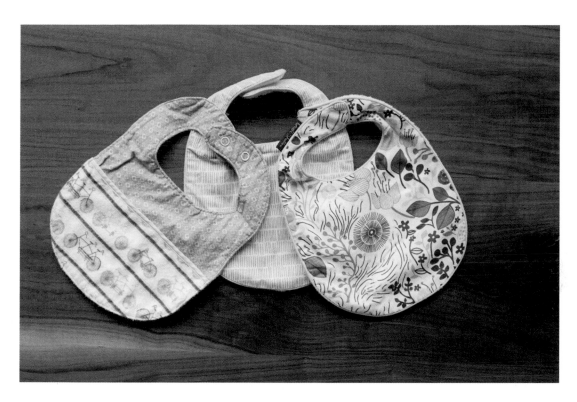

safety alert:
how to avoid choking

Once your baby starts eating finger foods, choking becomes more of a risk. Keep your little one safe by following these simple guidelines.

- Never leave your baby or toddler alone while he's eating, even if he seems well-practiced at finger foods.

- Make sure any finger foods that are small enough to fit into your baby's mouth (and not gnawed like a broccoli floret, cucumber strip, or watermelon wedge) are cut into tiny pieces, pea-sized or smaller. Round foods like grapes and hot dogs, in particular, should be sliced into small sections since they fit so neatly over a small child's windpipe.

- Avoid other common choking hazards like popcorn, whole nuts, spoonfuls of nut butter, hard candy, or soft, sticky foods like marshmallows or gummy candy.

- Be sure that all parents and caregivers are familiar with how to rescue a child if he does begin to choke. For details visit www.parents.com/choking.

BROCCOLI TREES WITH AVOCADO DIP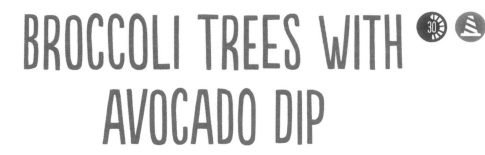

½ CUP BROCCOLI FLORETS

½ AVOCADO

2 TABLESPOONS PLAIN GREEK YOGURT

2 TABLESPOONS MAYONNAISE

1 TEASPOON LIME JUICE

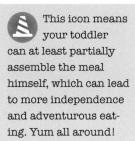 This icon means your toddler can at least partially assemble the meal himself, which can lead to more independence and adventurous eating. Yum all around!

Maximize your cooking time by steaming extra broccoli florets. Store them in the fridge for up to three days and serve later with more avocado dip, Spinach Pesto (see page 105), or toss in a salad.

1 In a medium saucepan, bring 2 inches of water to a simmer. Place a steamer basket over the water. Add the broccoli florets. Cover and steam until tender, about 5 minutes. Transfer to a plate.

2 Add the avocado, yogurt, mayonnaise, and lime juice to a food processor or blender. Process until smooth, adding a tablespoon or more water if needed to help it blend. Serve 2 tablespoons avocado dip with the broccoli.

Makes about ½ cup avocado dip

AGE IT UP: Add ¼ teaspoon salt and a few dashes of hot sauce to the avocado dip.

MAKE AHEAD: Both the broccoli florets and the dip keep well in the fridge for up to three days.

Nutrition per serving (2 tablespoons avocado dip and ¼ cup broccoli florets): 89 calories; 3g protein; 6g fat (1g sat. fat); 8g carbohydrates; 4g fiber; 2g sugars; 89mg sodium; 41mg calcium; 1mg iron; 326mg potassium; 52mg Vitamin C; 1247IU Vitamin A

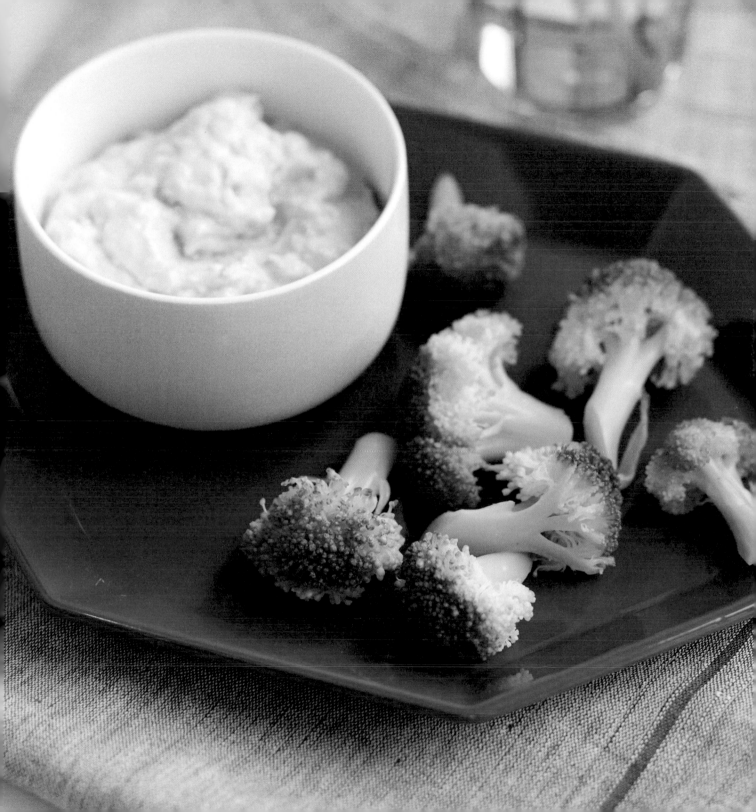

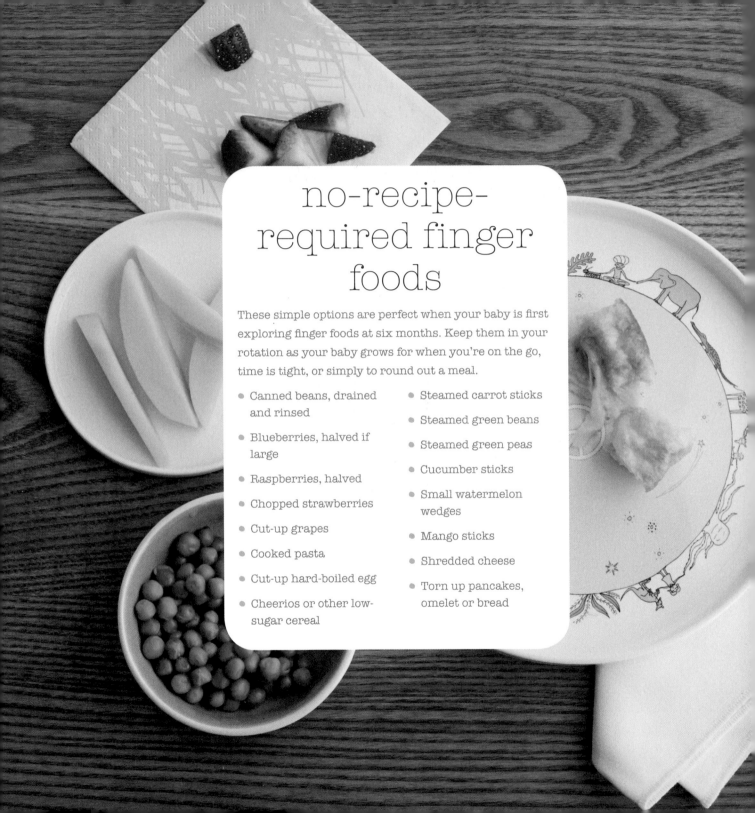

no-recipe-required finger foods

These simple options are perfect when your baby is first exploring finger foods at six months. Keep them in your rotation as your baby grows for when you're on the go, time is tight, or simply to round out a meal.

- Canned beans, drained and rinsed
- Blueberries, halved if large
- Raspberries, halved
- Chopped strawberries
- Cut-up grapes
- Cooked pasta
- Cut-up hard-boiled egg
- Cheerios or other low-sugar cereal
- Steamed carrot sticks
- Steamed green beans
- Steamed green peas
- Cucumber sticks
- Small watermelon wedges
- Mango sticks
- Shredded cheese
- Torn up pancakes, omelet or bread

SWEET-AND-SOUR TOFU STICKS

Introduce your baby to high-protein tofu at an early age and chances are this versatile, inexpensive, and nutritious ingredient will become one of your kitchen MVPs. These tofu sticks are delicious served warm, at room temperature, or straight from the fridge. They may seem a bit jiggly when fresh from the oven, but they'll firm up as they cool.

1 Place the tofu block on a plate lined with a few folded paper towels. Cover the tofu with more folded paper towels. Place another plate on top and weigh down the plate with something heavy, like a can of tomatoes. Let the tofu drain for 20 minutes. Slice the tofu into 12 sticks and transfer to a large, flat baking dish.

2 In a small bowl, whisk together the maple syrup, soy sauce, rice vinegar, and sesame oil. Pour over the tofu sticks and turn to coat. Let marinate for up to an hour, turning once.

3 Preheat the oven to 400°F. Line a rimmed baking sheet with parchment paper. Transfer the tofu sticks to the parchment paper, pouring any marinade over the top. Sprinkle with sesame seeds and bake for 30 minutes.

Makes 12 sticks

AGE IT UP: These tofu sticks have been a lunchbox staple in my house long beyond the finger food stage. They are also delicious chopped and added to salads or eaten plain as a simple snack.

Nutrition per serving (2 tofu sticks): 165 calories; 12g protein; 11g fat (2g sat. fat); 7g carbohydrates; 2g fiber; 3g sugars; 188mg sodium; 521mg calcium; 2mg iron; 191mg potassium; 0mg Vitamin C; 125IU Vitamin A

1 LB. EXTRA-FIRM TOFU, DRAINED

1 TABLESPOON MAPLE SYRUP

1 TABLESPOON LOW-SODIUM SOY SAUCE

1 TABLESPOON RICE VINEGAR

2 TABLESPOONS SESAME OIL

¼ TEASPOON SESAME SEEDS, WHITE OR BLACK

MAKE AHEAD: Keep the tofu sticks in the fridge for three to five days. Reheat them briefly in the microwave or a 250°F oven. Or, serve them cold or at room temperature.

SMOKY SQUASH CAKES

1 CUP BUTTERNUT SQUASH
PURÉE (SEE PAGE 40)

1 EGG, BEATEN

½ CUP PANKO BREADCRUMBS

1 SCALLION, FINELY
CHOPPED

2 TABLESPOONS CHOPPED
CILANTRO

¾ TEASPOON CUMIN

1 TABLESPOON OLIVE OIL,
PLUS MORE IF NECESSARY

Babies and toddlers will love this veggie pancake. Nutrition bonus: butternut squash is chock-full of vitamin A.

1 In a medium-sized bowl, combine all of the ingredients except for the olive oil. Form into 12 patties.

2 Heat 1 tablespoon olive oil in a large skillet over medium-high heat. Sauté the patties until golden brown, about 3 minutes per side, cooking in batches if necessary to avoid overcrowding.

Makes 12 patties

AGE IT UP: Add ¼ teaspoon salt to the batter. A little chopped jalapeño pepper would also be delicious.

MAKE AHEAD: Store in the fridge for up to three days. Serve at room temperature or reheat in a 250°F oven.

Nutrition per serving (2 patties): 80 calories; 2g protein; 3g fat (1g sat. fat); 10g carbohydrates; 1g fiber; 1g sugars; 78mg sodium; 36mg calcium; 1mg iron; 139mg potassium; 7mg Vitamin C; 3370IU Vitamin A

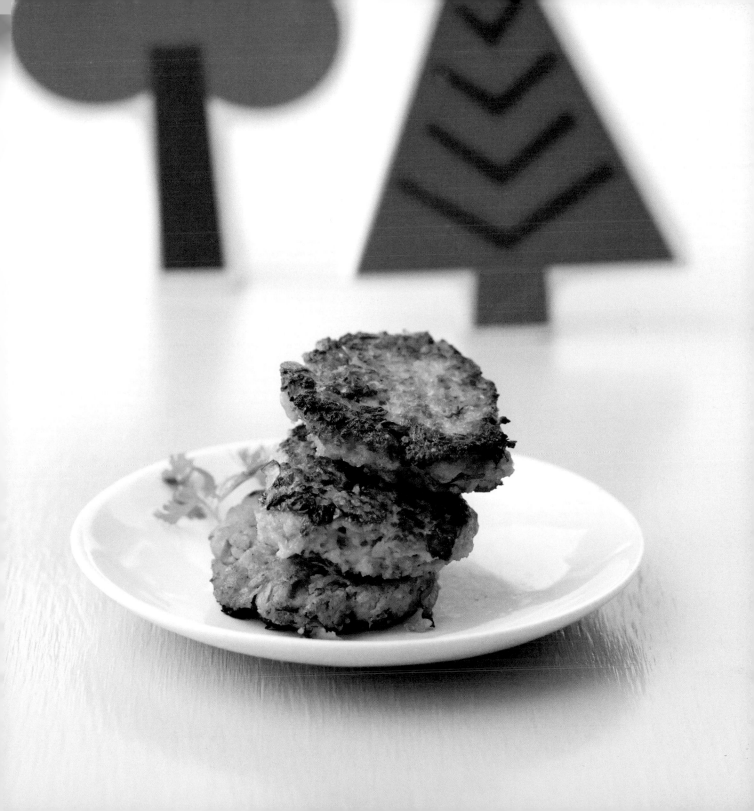

MAPLE GRAHAM ANIMALS

½ CUP WHOLE-WHEAT
GRAHAM FLOUR OR WHOLE-
WHEAT FLOUR

½ CUP ALL-PURPOSE FLOUR,
PLUS MORE FOR DUSTING

½ TEASPOON BAKING
POWDER

½ TEASPOON CINNAMON

⅛ TEASPOON SALT

¼ CUP UNSALTED BUTTER,
SOFTENED

2 TABLESPOONS MILK

2 TABLESPOONS MAPLE
SYRUP

Skip the trans fat and high-fructose corn syrup found in many processed animal crackers. Mix up this lightly sweetened whole-grain dough instead and cut away. Animal-shaped crackers are cute, but little circles and stars also delight.

1 Preheat the oven to 375°F. Line a rimmed baking sheet with parchment paper.

2 In a large bowl, whisk together the two flours, baking powder, cinnamon, and salt. Using an electric mixer, beat in the butter, milk, and maple syrup just until a stiff dough forms.

3 Sprinkle a clean work surface with flour. Transfer the dough to the work surface and roll it out to ¼-inch thickness. Using small cookie cutters (about 1½ inches wide), cut shapes from the dough and place them on the baking sheet. Re-roll and cut the remaining dough. Bake for 12 to 14 minutes or until golden brown.

Makes about 60 small crackers

MAKE AHEAD: Keep the animal crackers in an airtight container at room temperature for up to five days.

Nutrition per serving (6 crackers): 93 calories; 1g protein; 5g fat (3g sat. fat); 12g carbohydrates; 1g fiber; 3g sugars; 31mg sodium; 21mg calcium; 1mg iron; 66mg potassium; 0mg Vitamin C; 143IU Vitamin A

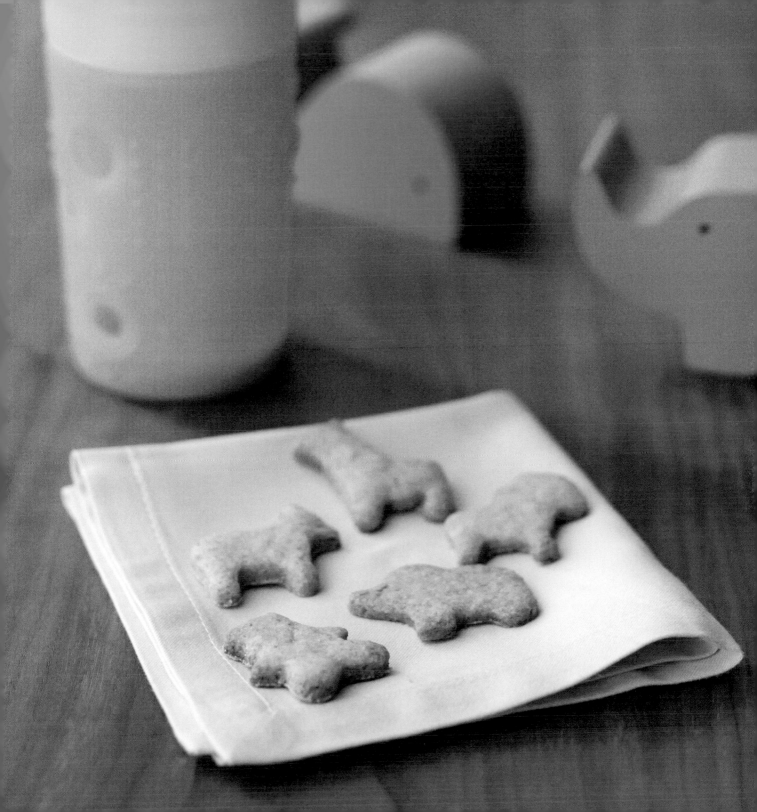

MISO-SESAME SWEET POTATOES

3 LARGE SWEET POTATOES

⅓ CUP WHITE MISO PASTE

⅔ CUP TAHINI (SESAME SEED PASTE)

¾ CUP WATER

¼ CUP APPLE JUICE

3 TABLESPOONS MAPLE SYRUP

MISO

Miso is a savory paste made from fermented soybeans that is available in the refrigerated section at better-stocked grocery stores. Whenever possible, look to add more fermented foods like kimchi, traditional pickles, sauerkraut, and miso to your family's diet. They are packed with digestion-friendly probiotics that promote good gut health.

These sweet potato wedges are faintly sweet, nutty, and mellow—a real crowd pleaser. The addictive glaze keeps forever, so consider making a double batch and saving some to use on fish, whisk into salad dressing, top simple steamed vegetables, or sneak straight from the spoon…you'll see.

1 Preheat the oven to 400°F. Line a rimmed baking sheet with parchment paper.

2 Cut the sweet potatoes into ½-inch thick wedges and set aside in a large bowl.

3 In a small bowl, combine the miso, tahini, water, apple juice, and maple syrup and whisk until completely blended. Pour about half of the miso mixture over the sweet potatoes and toss to coat evenly.

4 Lay the potatoes in a single layer on the prepared baking sheet. Roast for 40 to 45 minutes, until browned. Serve warm or at room temperature, with extra sauce drizzled on top or served on the side as a dip.

Makes about 8 servings

MAKE AHEAD: Store the roasted sweet potatoes in the refrigerator for up to three days. Reheat in a 250°F oven until warm.

Nutrition per serving (¼ cup sweet potato wedges): 213 calories; 6g protein; 10g fat (1g sat. fat); 28g carbohydrates; 5g fiber; 10g sugars; 466mg sodium; 119mg calcium; 1mg iron; 446mg potassium; 13mg Vitamin C; 12994IU Vitamin A

CORNMEAL and ZUCCHINI PANCAKES

Serve these wholesome pancakes with Greek yogurt, sour cream, or applesauce for dipping.

1 Wrap the grated zucchini in a clean towel, and squeeze out as much moisture as possible.

2 In a large bowl, combine the zucchini, scallions, eggs, cheese, milk, and pepper to taste. In a small bowl, stir together the cornmeal and baking powder. Add the dry ingredients to the zucchini mixture and stir to combine.

3 Heat 1 tablespoon of olive oil in a large skillet over medium-high heat. When the oil is hot, drop the batter into the pan by the tablespoonful. Cook for about 3 minutes on the first side, until the pancakes start to look set around the edges and the bottoms are golden. Flip and cook for about 2 minutes more. Place the cooked pancakes on a paper towel-lined plate and repeat with the remaining oil and batter.

Makes about 24 pancakes

AGE IT UP: Add 1 teaspoon salt to the batter.

MAKE AHEAD: These pancakes keep well in the fridge for up to three days. When you're ready to serve again, simply spread them out on a tray in a 250°F oven until they're warm and crisp.

2 LARGE ZUCCHINI, GRATED (ABOUT 5 CUPS)

¼ CUP FINELY CHOPPED SCALLIONS

2 LARGE EGGS

1½ CUPS SHREDDED CHEDDAR CHEESE

¾ CUP MILK

FRESHLY GROUND PEPPER, TO TASTE

2 CUPS CORNMEAL

1 TEASPOON BAKING POWDER

2 TABLESPOONS OLIVE OIL

Nutrition per serving (2 pancakes): 208 calories; 8g protein; 9g fat (4g sat. fat); 24g carbohydrates; 2g fiber; 3g sugars; 146mg sodium; 164mg calcium; 2mg iron; 231mg potassium; 10mg Vitamin C; 4017IU Vitamin A

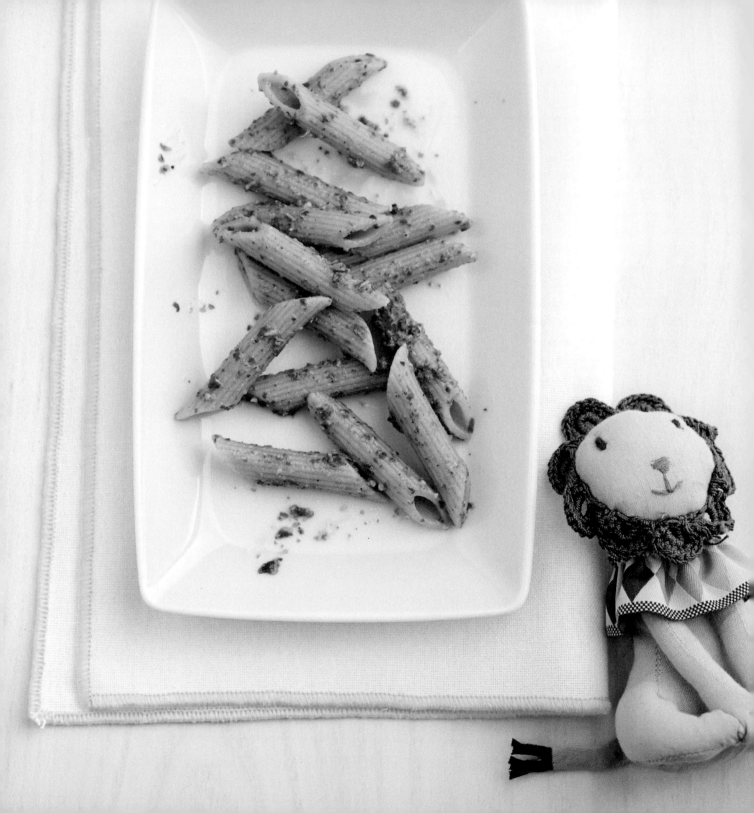

PASTA *with* SPINACH PESTO

Mark this recipe. You'll want to make this pesto long after your little one is past the finger food stage.

1 Bring a medium pot of water to a boil. Add the spinach and cook for 15 seconds. Drain well, squeezing out any water with a fork.

2 Add all of the pesto ingredients, including the spinach, to a food processor and process until smooth. To serve, mix 2 teaspoons pesto with ¼ cup cooked pasta, or serve the pesto as a dip.

Makes 1 cup pesto

AGE IT UP: Add ¼ teaspoon salt to the pesto, plus more to taste.

MAKE AHEAD: Transfer the pesto to a storage container, cover with a thin layer of olive oil, and refrigerate for up to three days. Bring to room temperature for 15 minutes before serving. Or, transfer to multiple small containers (so you can defrost just as much as you need), cover with a thin layer of oil, and freeze.

For pesto:

ONE 5-OZ. PACKAGE BABY SPINACH

2 CUPS BASIL, PACKED

¼ CUP WALNUTS, LIGHTLY TOASTED

¼ CUP GRATED PARMESAN CHEESE

1 SMALL CLOVE GARLIC

½ CUP OLIVE OIL

For serving:

¼ CUP COOKED WHOLE-GRAIN PENNE PASTA

Nutrition per serving (¼ cup whole-grain pasta with 2 teaspoons pesto): 96 calories; 3g protein; 6g fat (1g sat. fat); 10g carbohydrates; 1g fiber; 0g sugars; 22mg sodium; 27mg calcium; 1mg iron; 61mg potassium; 2mg Vitamin C; 668IU Vitamin A

POLENTA DIAMONDS

1½ CUPS WATER

½ CUP QUICK-COOKING POLENTA

1 TABLESPOON UNSALTED BUTTER

For serving:

¼ CUP GO-TO TOMATO SAUCE (SEE PAGE 191)

These chubby sticks are easy for little hands to pick up and dunk into tangy tomato sauce.

1 In a medium saucepan over high heat, bring the water to a boil. Pour in the polenta in a smooth stream, whisking all the while to prevent lumps. Turn the heat to low and simmer the polenta until thickened and smooth, 3 to 5 minutes, stirring frequently.

2 Fit a large piece of parchment paper into an 8 x 8 baking dish, leaving the parchment overhanging the sides like handles. Pour the polenta into the dish, spreading it with a spatula until even. Let cool for 30 minutes.

3 Preheat the oven to 350°F. Lift the parchment out of the baking dish and place it on a cutting board. Cut the polenta into 12 diamonds or rectangles. Transfer the parchment to a baking sheet. Spread out the diamonds and bake for 10 minutes.

4 Serve the diamonds with Go-To Tomato Sauce for dipping.

Makes 12 diamonds

AGE IT UP: Add ¼ teaspoon salt to the polenta as it cooks.

MAKE AHEAD: Keep the polenta in the fridge for up to three days. Reheat briefly in the microwave or a 250°F oven. Or serve the diamonds cold or at room temperature.

Nutrition per serving (2 diamonds and ¼ cup dipping sauce): 112 calories; 2g protein; 5g fat (3g sat. fat); 16g carbohydrates; 2g fiber; 4g sugars; 222mg sodium; 28mg calcium; 1mg iron; 252mg potassium; 7mg Vitamin C; 712IU Vitamin A

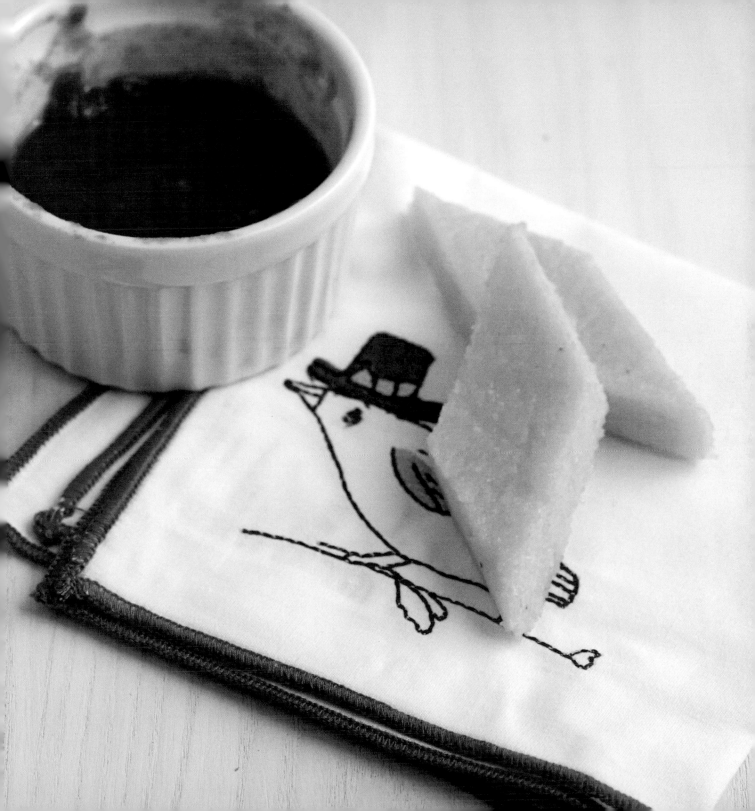

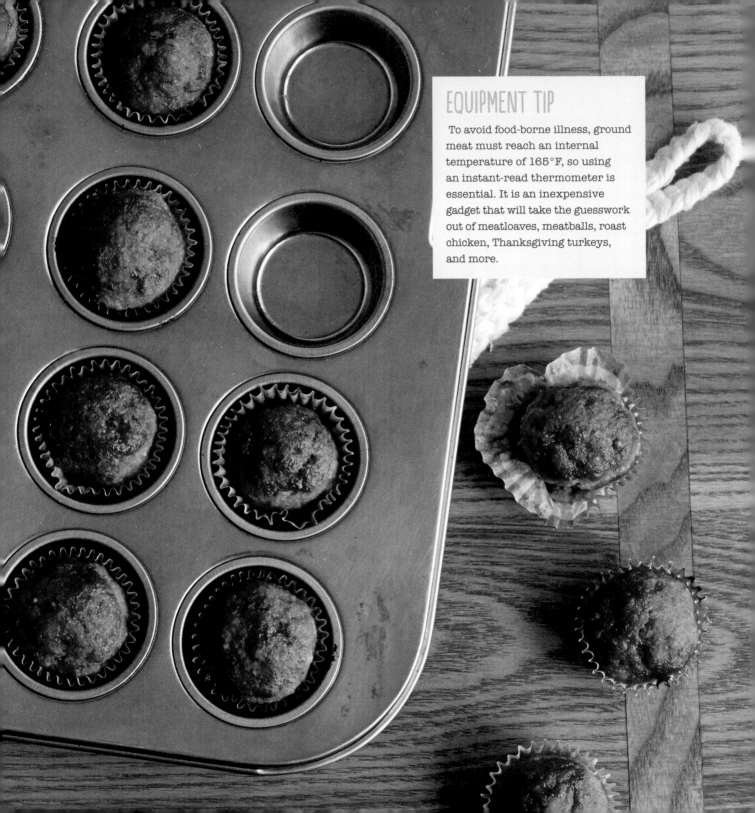

EQUIPMENT TIP

To avoid food-borne illness, ground meat must reach an internal temperature of 165°F, so using an instant-read thermometer is essential. It is an inexpensive gadget that will take the guesswork out of meatloaves, meatballs, roast chicken, Thanksgiving turkeys, and more.

Mini Maple BBQ
TURKEY MEATLOAF BITES

This recipe comes from my friend and fellow personal chef Suzy Scherr. Her little ones love these fun-sized meatloaves, which pack lots of protein in a tiny package. Any ground meat works here, so use whichever your family likes best.

1 Preheat the oven to 350°F. Lightly grease a 24-cup mini muffin pan with cooking spray or insert liners.

2 In a small bowl, make the BBQ sauce by combining the ketchup, maple syrup, vinegar, Worcestershire, paprika, and cayenne, if using. Mix well and set aside.

3 Crack the egg in a large bowl and beat it with a fork. Add the ground turkey, breadcrumbs, onion and garlic powders, and half the BBQ sauce. Mix well. Divide the turkey mixture evenly among the muffin cups. Brush the tops with the remaining BBQ sauce.

4 Bake for 25 to 30 minutes or until the internal temperature of each meatloaf reaches 165°F when tested with an instant-read thermometer.

Makes 24 meatloaves

MAKE AHEAD: Store the meatloaves in the fridge in an airtight container for up to three days. Reheat in a 250°F oven or the microwave until warm. Meatloaves are also tasty at room temperature.

⅔ CUP KETCHUP

6 TABLESPOONS MAPLE SYRUP

1½ TABLESPOONS WHITE WINE VINEGAR

1½ TABLESPOONS WORCESTERSHIRE SAUCE

2 TEASPOONS PAPRIKA

PINCH CAYENNE (OPTIONAL)

1 EGG

1 LB. GROUND TURKEY (PREFERABLY 94% LEAN)

½ CUP DRIED BREADCRUMBS

1 TABLESPOON ONION POWDER

1 TABLESPOON GARLIC POWDER

Nutrition per serving (2 meatloaves): 137 calories; 8g protein; 5g fat (2g sat. fat); 15g carbohydrates; 1g fiber; 10g sugars; 230mg sodium; 41mg calcium; 1mg iron; 204mg potassium; 2mg Vitamin C; 372IU Vitamin A

Should Your Baby Go Gluten-Free?

It's no surprise that many parents are asking themselves this question. With so much media attention given to gluten-free diets, it's tempting to believe that delaying its introduction to your baby or avoiding it altogether will help prevent celiac disease or other gluten-related disorders. But chances are, that's not the case.

What is gluten and is it harmful for your baby? Gluten is a type of plant protein found in some grains like wheat, barley, and rye. It is also a common food additive used to improve the texture of a variety of processed foods from deli meats to ketchup. Some children develop an autoimmune reaction to gluten called celiac disease and need to avoid it even in the smallest amounts since consumption of gluten leads to intestinal damage and compromised absorption of nutrients. As a result, these children may develop symptoms like gas, intestinal pain, constipation, diarrhea, or weight loss, and long-term health complications like osteoporosis, neurological problems, and anemia. Celiac disease can be diagnosed with a blood test and endoscopy. Avoiding gluten is the only treatment available currently.

Another gluten related disorder, non-celiac gluten sensitivity, does not produce antibodies and intestinal damage and cannot be diagnosed with the same tests, but it triggers similar symptoms that resolve once gluten has been removed from the diet.

Finally, an allergy to wheat can be diagnosed with skin prick tests, wheat-specific IgE blood testing, and a clinical food challenge. It is also managed by removing gluten-containing foods from the diet since the allergic reaction is triggered by exposure to wheat proteins. Some signs of wheat allergy include abdominal pain, nausea, vomiting, diarrhea, skin rashes, runny nose, and conjunctivitis.

If you suspect that your child has celiac disease, non-celiac gluten sensitivity, or a wheat allergy, make sure to discuss relevant tests with your doctor. You may also need to speak to a dietitian to help you follow a restrictive wheat or gluten-free diet while meeting your child's nutritional needs.

Should healthy kids avoid gluten? Gluten is harmless for the vast majority of children who do not have any symptoms of gluten-related disorders. In fact, avoiding it may lead to insufficient intake of certain nutrients, such as B vitamins and iron, found in fortified wheat products like breads and cereals. Besides, although many gluten-free products have a "health halo", they may have more added sugars and fat than their wheat counterparts and cost more money to boot.

When is the best time to introduce gluten into your baby's diet? The American Academy of Pediatrics has not released any official recommendations concerning the timing of introduction of gluten in order to cut the risk of gluten intolerance in the future. Neither introducing gluten early nor delaying its introduction seems to help prevent celiac disease in the future. So the short answer is, introduce it whenever you want, but know that for most babies there is no reason to wait.

If you have a strong history of gluten intolerance in your family, make sure to talk to your doctor to discuss the best way to introduce gluten into your baby's diet. If gluten is safe for your baby, but you still feel it is best to avoid it, make sure to explore a wide selection of gluten-free whole grains such as quinoa, millet, rice, teff, buckwheat, amaranth, and corn rather than stocking up on gluten-free processed treats like cookies and granola bars. Strive to eat whole foods free of gluten, not gluten-free processed foods.

- Natalia Stasenko, MS, RD

chapter five

WAKE-UP TIME

NUTRITIOUS BREAKFASTS FOR A HAPPY, HEALTHY MORNING
(12 months and up)

I discovered early on that the best way to get Rosa out of bed is the promise of breakfast. Whether peanut butter on cinnamon raisin bread, egg on a whole wheat bagel, pancakes, French toast, or a frittata, breakfast food is universally adored at my house. When I was growing up, though, my mother rarely ate traditional breakfast food in the morning. Instead, she heated up leftovers from dinner the night before, ate cheese and crackers, or sprinkled lima beans with Parmesan cheese. As a child I thought it was more than bizarre. But now I say to each her own and a happy, healthy breakfast to all.

Most weekdays my breakfast strategy is all about speed, so I will put something together in under five minutes, such as a 60-Second Egg (see page 115) and Avocado Toast (see page 123). Or I'll spend a little more time on the weekend making a batch of muffins or pancakes I can call into action on a moment's notice. Either way, I've got an eager kid at the table ready to start the day.

a breakfast of champions (a.k.a. toddlers)

Good morning! While you may be bleary-eyed before that first cup of coffee has kicked in, toddlers are not only hungry when they wake up, they are often in the best mood of the day, and more open to trying new flavors. Take advantage and offer little ones a healthy, delicious meal that will both energize them and expand their palates.

But serving breakfast can be full of pitfalls. Mornings are so busy that sometimes it seems easier to just pour a "healthy" cereal or zap an often heavily sweetened pack of instant oatmeal in the microwave. Some breakfast must be better than no breakfast, right?

Well, yes, but...we can do better. The recipes in this chapter were created with the realities of modern breakfast in mind. They all come together in 15 minutes or (much) less, or can easily be made ahead of time. Leftovers can be saved for weekdays or even frozen. The chapter progresses from super-simple recipes to ones requiring a bit more prep.

So give your kiddo a healthy, wholesome start to the day with quality proteins and fats, fruits, and even vegetables, without the scads of added sugars typically found in packaged breakfast cereals, bars, or drinks. She'll be happier, healthier, and ready to face a busy day of playing, sleeping, growing, and learning.

60-SECOND EGG

Balanced sources of protein and healthy fats, eggs are one of nature's most perfect foods. For a complete breakfast, serve one egg with toast triangles and a bit of fruit.

1 Lightly grease a 4-ounce ramekin or small bowl with butter or olive oil. Crack the egg into the ramekin. Sprinkle in salt and pepper to taste, and stir with a fork.

2 Cover with a paper towel and microwave for 45 to 60 seconds, depending on the level of doneness you prefer. Take care removing the ramekin from the microwave, since it will be hot. Using a fork, gently transfer the egg to a plate, cool briefly, and serve.

Makes 1 egg

UNSALTED BUTTER OR OLIVE OIL FOR GREASING THE RAMEKIN

1 EGG

PINCH SALT

FRESHLY GROUND PEPPER, TO TASTE

Nutrition per serving: 83 calories; 6g protein; 6g fat (2g sat. fat); 0g carbohydrates; 0g fiber; 0g sugars; 218mg sodium; 25mg calcium; 1mg iron; 61mg potassium; 0mg Vitamin C; 238IU Vitamin A

SOAKED OATS (A.K.A. MUESLI)

Muesli:

1¾ CUPS ROLLED OATS

¼ CUP RAW, UNSALTED SUNFLOWER SEEDS

¼ CUP FINELY CHOPPED PECANS

¼ CUP CHOPPED PITTED PRUNES

¼ CUP CHOPPED DRIED CHERRIES

PINCH SALT

For serving:

½ CUP MUESLI

¼ CUP PLAIN GREEK YOGURT

¼ CUP MILK

½ TEASPOON HONEY OR MAPLE SYRUP

Oats become tender, creamy, and downright luscious when soaked overnight in milk and yogurt—no cooking required! Make sure to use rolled oats, not instant, and feel free to sub in whichever nuts or dried fruits you have on hand.

1 In a medium bowl, combine the oats, sunflower seeds, pecans, prunes, cherries, and salt.

2 The night before serving, stir together ½ cup of the muesli, the yogurt, and milk. Cover and store in the refrigerator overnight. Drizzle with honey or maple syrup and serve.

Makes about 3½ cups

MAKE AHEAD: Store the muesli at room temperature in an airtight container for up to two weeks.

WHOLESOME TIP

Between the ages of one and two, toddlers should eat energy-rich, full-fat milk and yogurt. Once they reach age two they can transition to reduced-fat or low-fat dairy products.

Nutrition per serving with full-fat dairy (¼ cup): 294 calories; 13g protein; 12g fat (4g sat. fat); 35g carbohydrates; 4g fiber; 12g sugars; 76mg sodium; 145mg calcium; 2mg iron; 190mg potassium; 1mg Vitamin C; 229IU Vitamin A

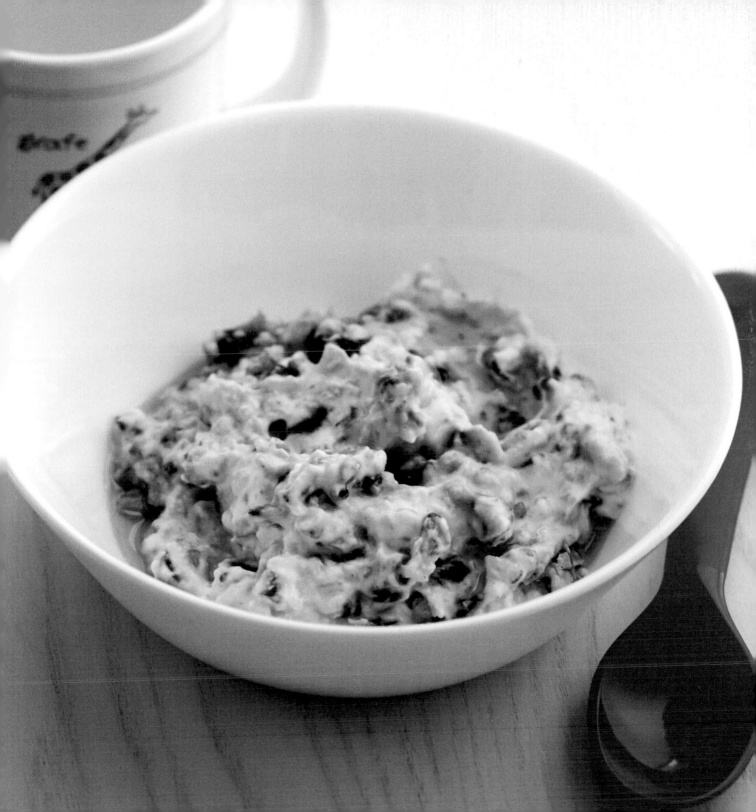

BLUEBERRY-SPINACH SHAKE

⅓ CUP MILK

½ BANANA

½ CUP PACKED BABY SPINACH

½ CUP FROZEN BLUEBERRIES

1 TABLESPOON GROUND FLAXSEEDS

Add some veg to breakfast with this sweet, satisfying smoothie. Feel free to use unsweetened almond milk or soy milk for a vegan version. By 12 months most toddlers should be able to use an open cup to slurp up a smoothie. Straw cups are another—less messy—option.

Add all of the ingredients to the blender, beginning with the milk. Cover and blend until smooth, about 30 seconds.

Makes 1 serving

WHOLESOME TIP

Flaxseeds are high in fiber, a good source of plant omega-3 fatty acids, and a source of beneficial phytochemicals called lignans. They are also mild in flavor and play well with a multitude of other foods. Sprinkle flax on oatmeal, stir into muffin batter, or blend into any smoothie for an extra nutritional boost. Make sure to buy ground flaxseeds, as whole flaxseeds are not digestible, and store them in the fridge for freshness.

Nutrition per serving with full-fat dairy (1 smoothie): 191 calories; 6g protein; 6g fat (2g sat. fat); 31g carbohydrates; 6g fiber; 15g sugars; 66mg sodium; 150mg calcium; 2mg iron; 449mg potassium; 21mg Vitamin C; 2025IU Vitamin A

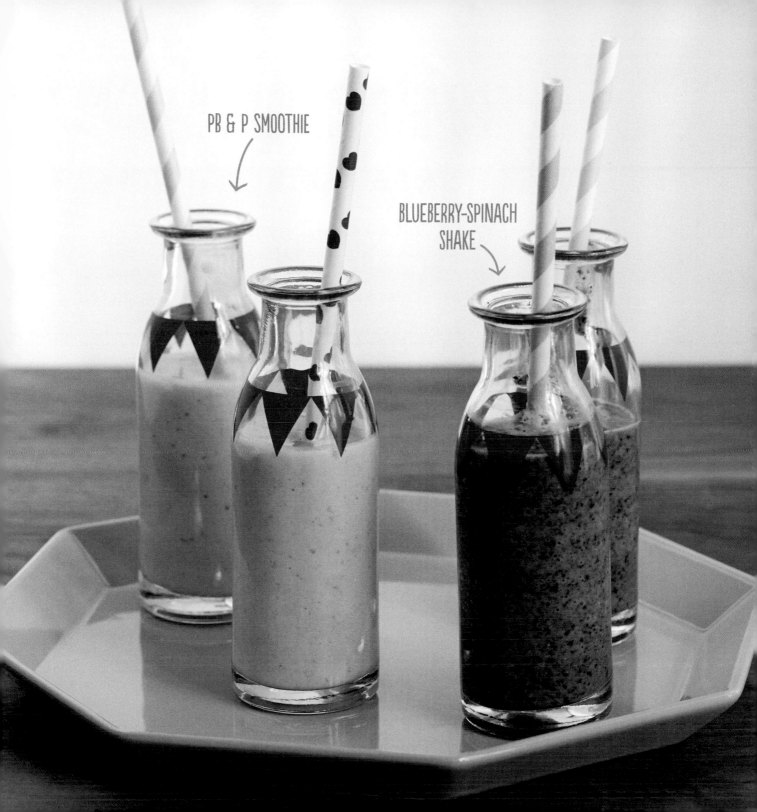

PB & P SMOOTHIE

BLUEBERRY-SPINACH
SHAKE

PB & P SMOOTHIE

½ CUP MILK

½ BANANA

½ CUP FROZEN SLICED PEACHES

1 TABLESPOON CREAMY PEANUT BUTTER, PREFERABLY UNSWEETENED

This naturally sweet smoothie is packed with protein thanks to the milk and peanut butter, and potassium courtesy of the banana. Almond butter or sunflower seed butter stand in nicely for the peanut butter, if you prefer, and any frozen fruit can sub for the peaches. Frozen strawberries or grapes make for an especially appealing flavor combination.

Add all of the ingredients to the blender, beginning with the milk. Cover and blend until smooth, about 30 seconds.

Makes 1 serving

Nutrition per serving with full-fat dairy (1 smoothie): 253 calories; 9g protein; 13g fat (4g sat. fat); 30g carbohydrates; 4g fiber; 15g sugars; 67mg sodium; 166mg calcium; 1mg iron; 546mg potassium; 12mg Vitamin C; 461IU Vitamin A

Double Almond
QUINOA PORRIDGE

This creamy porridge is a comforting breakfast on a cold morning. It's also a smart use for leftover quinoa, that protein-packed seed that's synonymous with healthy eating these days, and rightly so.

Combine the quinoa, almond butter, almond milk, and maple syrup in a small saucepan over medium heat. Stir until the almond butter has melted into the quinoa and the porridge is warmed through. Transfer to a bowl and sprinkle with cinnamon.

Makes 1 serving

½ CUP COOKED QUINOA

1 TABLESPOON UNSWEETENED ALMOND BUTTER

¼ CUP UNSWEETENED ALMOND MILK

½ TEASPOON MAPLE SYRUP

CINNAMON, FOR SPRINKLING

Nutrition per serving: 228 calories; 8g protein; 11g fat (1g sat. fat); 25g carbohydrates; 5g fiber; 3g sugars; 53mg sodium; 125mg calcium; 2mg iron; 333mg potassium; 0mg Vitamin C; 130IU Vitamin A

TOPPINGS *for* TOAST

Breakfast doesn't get much easier than these. Simply toast a slice of whole-wheat or sprouted bread, mash one of these fillings, and spread on the toast for a filling, nutritious meal.

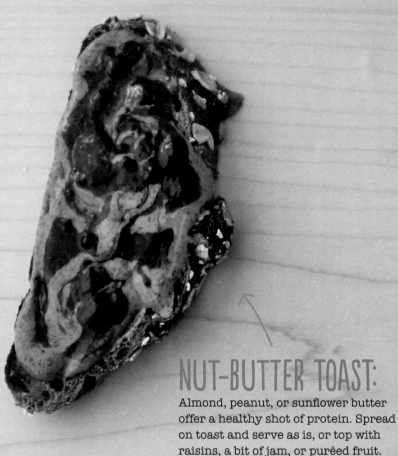

NUT-BUTTER TOAST:

Almond, peanut, or sunflower butter offer a healthy shot of protein. Spread on toast and serve as is, or top with raisins, a bit of jam, or puréed fruit.

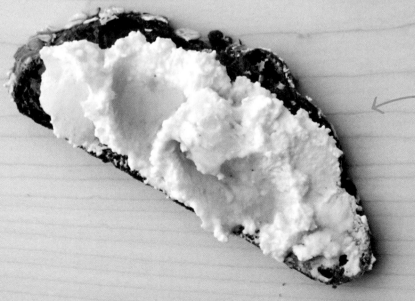

RICOTTA-HONEY TOAST:

Creamy ricotta spreads like a dream. Sprinkle with lemon zest and drizzle with honey for a flavorful breakfast.

EGG-YOGURT TOAST:

Chop a hard-boiled egg, smash with a tablespoon of plain yogurt and a pinch of salt, and serve on toast.

AVOCADO TOAST:

Mash ½ ripe avocado in a small bowl with a fork until smooth. Spread on the toast. Sprinkle with a bit of salt and drizzle with a squeeze of lemon or lime juice.

WHOLESOME TIP

Make sure the sliced bread you keep on hand is made with whole grains. Many front-of-package claims can be misleading, so skip right to the ingredient list. The word "whole" should be the first word on the list, and each slice of bread should have at least 3 grams of fiber and 1 gram of sugar or less. Another smart option is sprouted bread. Often found in the freezer section of the supermarket, this bread isn't made from regular flour, but instead from nutrient-packed sprouted grains. If sprouted bread is made with legumes like beans and lentils, it provides complete proteins (rare for plant-based foods). Another perk: sprouted breads typically contain little or no sugar.

123

BREAKFAST FRIED RICE

2 TEASPOONS CANOLA OIL

½ CUP COOKED BROWN RICE, COLD

½ CUP FINELY CHOPPED COOKED BROCCOLI

1 EGG, BEATEN

1 TEASPOON LOW-SODIUM SOY SAUCE

This savory breakfast comes together in five minutes and is an excellent way to clean out the fridge. Use virtually any vegetable you have on hand; frozen and thawed peas are another toddler-friendly option. While brown rice is best nutrition-wise, white will work in a pinch.

1 Heat the oil in a medium nonstick skillet over medium-high heat. Add the brown rice and broccoli. Sauté, stirring frequently, for 2 minutes.

2 Using a spoon, clear a space in the center of the pan. Add the egg and stir to scramble, incorporating the rice and broccoli. Add the soy sauce and continue stirring until the egg is fully cooked. Serve immediately.

Makes 1 serving

Nutrition per serving: 282 calories; 10g protein; 14g fat (2g sat. fat); 29g carbohydrates; 4g fiber; 1g sugars; 272mg sodium; 66mg calcium; 2mg iron; 375mg potassium; 51mg Vitamin C; 1445IU Vitamin A

TROPICAL TOAST

French toast is one of the few weekend favorites that is also weekday-workable. Cooked French toast can be kept warm in a 200°F oven for up to 30 minutes. Saucy Fruit (see page 129) also makes a delightful topping for this toast.

1 In a large dish, beat the egg, coconut milk, agave nectar, and vanilla until combined.

2 Heat a large griddle or nonstick skillet over medium heat. Brush with a bit of canola oil. Dip the bread slices into the egg mixture. Fry the bread in a single layer until golden brown, about 3 minutes per side, cooking in batches if necessary to avoid overcrowding.

3 Sprinkle the French toast with lime zest, if using, and serve with a bit of maple syrup.

Makes 4 slices

MAKE AHEAD: Refrigerate for up to three days and reheat in the microwave, oven, or toaster.

EQUIPMENT TIP: If you plan on making pancakes or French toast regularly I highly recommend buying a flat griddle that covers two burners. It will slash your cooking time and should cost about $60 at a cooking supply store or online. I shudder to think of the hours of my life I lost flipping two pancakes at a time in a frying pan during my pre-griddle days.

1 EGG

½ CUP COCONUT MILK (REFRIGERATED, NOT CANNED) OR COW'S MILK

1½ TEASPOONS AGAVE NECTAR

½ TEASPOON VANILLA EXTRACT

CANOLA OIL, FOR THE GRIDDLE

4 SLICES WHOLE-GRAIN OR SPROUTED BREAD

LIME ZEST (OPTIONAL) AND MAPLE SYRUP FOR SERVING

Nutrition per serving (1 slice): 165 calories; 5g protein; 5g fat (1g sat. fat); 27g carbohydrates; 3g fiber; 5g sugars; 176mg sodium; 33mg calcium; 2mg iron; 170mg potassium; 0mg Vitamin C; 122IU Vitamin A

PUMPKIN SPICE PANCAKES

1 CUP COCONUT OR
COW'S MILK

2 TABLESPOONS
COCONUT OIL, MELTED,
OR CANOLA OIL

1 EGG

1 TEASPOON VANILLA
EXTRACT

¾ CUP ALL-PURPOSE FLOUR

½ CUP WHOLE-WHEAT
FLOUR

1 TABLESPOON SUGAR

2 TEASPOONS BAKING
POWDER

1½ TEASPOONS CINNAMON

¼ TEASPOON SALT

½ CUP PUMPKIN PURÉE

CANOLA OIL, FOR THE
GRIDDLE

These fluffy, delicious pancakes are so good, you'll want to eat them for breakfast, lunch, and dinner. Pumpkin purée gives them a boost of vitamin A.

1 In a large bowl, whisk together the milk, coconut oil, egg, and vanilla. Add the two flours, sugar, baking powder, cinnamon, and salt, and stir to combine. Stir in the pumpkin purée.

2 Heat a griddle or nonstick skillet over medium heat and brush with a bit of canola oil. Drop the pancake batter by ¼-cupfuls onto the griddle. Cook until the edges seem dry, about 3 minutes. Flip and cook for 2 more minutes or until the pancakes are cooked through.

Makes about 12 pancakes

MAKE AHEAD: Refrigerate for up to three days and reheat in the microwave, oven, or toaster. Freeze pancakes in a zip-top bag separated by sheets of parchment or waxed paper. Defrost in the microwave or toaster.

WHOLESOME TIP

Coconut milk and coconut oil add a lovely, warm flavor to these scrumptious pancakes. Skip canned coconut milk, which is much higher in fat and calories, and look for coconut milk in cartons near the refrigerated soy milk or shelf-stable almond milk. Coconut oil is worth having in your pantry as a non-dairy substitute for butter in baked goods and a flavorful fat for Asian-style dishes.

Nutrition per pancake: 88 calories; 2g protein; 4g fat (3g sat. fat); 12g carbohydrates; 1g fiber; 2g sugars; 116mg sodium; 72mg calcium; 1mg iron; 60mg potassium; 0mg Vitamin C; 1650IU Vitamin A

GREEK YOGURT PANCAKES

Greek yogurt, flax, and whole-wheat flour add extra nutritional punch to these toddler- (and teen and grown-up…) pleasing pancakes.

1. In a large bowl, whisk together the egg, milk, and yogurt. Add the two flours, flax, sugar, baking powder, baking soda, and salt, and stir to combine.

2. Heat a griddle or large nonstick skillet over medium heat and brush with a bit of canola oil. Drop the pancake batter by ¼ cupfuls onto the griddle. Cook until the edges seem dry, about 3 minutes. Flip and cook for 2 more minutes or until the pancakes are cooked through.

Makes about 10 pancakes

MAKE AHEAD: Refrigerate for up to three days and reheat in the microwave, oven, or toaster. Freeze pancakes in a zip-top bag separated by sheets of parchment or waxed paper. Defrost in the microwave or toaster.

1 EGG

½ CUP MILK

½ CUP PLAIN GREEK YOGURT

½ CUP ALL-PURPOSE FLOUR

¼ CUP PLUS 2 TABLESPOONS WHOLE-WHEAT FLOUR

2 TABLESPOONS GROUND FLAXSEEDS

2 TABLESPOONS SUGAR

¾ TEASPOON BAKING POWDER

¼ TEASPOON BAKING SODA

¼ TEASPOON SALT

CANOLA OIL, FOR THE GRIDDLE

Nutrition per pancake: 81 calories; 4g protein; 2g fat (1g sat. fat); 12g carbohydrates; 1g fiber; 3g sugars; 138mg sodium; 65mg calcium; 0mg iron; 64mg potassium; 0mg Vitamin C; 54IU Vitamin A

BAKED PANCAKE *with* SAUCY FRUIT

2 EGGS

1½ CUPS MILK

1 TEASPOON VANILLA

¾ CUP FLOUR

3 TABLESPOONS SUGAR

½ TEASPOON SALT

2 TABLESPOONS UNSALTED BUTTER

2 CUPS SAUCY FRUIT

When I was a kid my mom made a delicious, buttery baked pancake. And when I say buttery, I mean it. That puffy pancake virtually swam in butter. This version is much less greasy, but still golden and custard-y. Sure, you could top it with maple syrup, but juicy fruit is just as sweet and much more nutritious.

1 Preheat the oven to 450°F. Place a 10-inch heavy skillet or pie plate into the oven.

2 In a medium bowl, whisk together the eggs, milk, vanilla, flour, sugar, and salt.

3 Carefully add the butter to the hot pan in the oven. Close the oven door and let the butter melt and turn a light (not dark!) brown, 1 to 2 minutes. Remove the pan from the oven and add the batter.

4 Return the pan to the oven and cook until golden and set, about 20 minutes. Let stand at room temperature for 5 minutes (the pancake will deflate a bit), cut into wedges, and serve with Saucy Fruit.

Makes about 4 servings

Nutrition per serving (pancake only): 262 calories; 9g protein; 10g fat (6g sat. fat); 34g carbohydrates; 1g fiber; 11g sugars; 370mg sodium; 131mg calcium; 2mg iron; 201mg potassium; 1mg Vitamin C; 486IU Vitamin A

Nutrition per serving (⅓ cup Saucy Fruit): 32 calories; 1g protein; 0g fat (0g sat. fat); 8g carbohydrates; 2g fiber; 6g sugars; 1mg sodium; 12mg calcium; 0mg iron; 116mg potassium; 44mg Vitamin C; 9IU Vitamin A

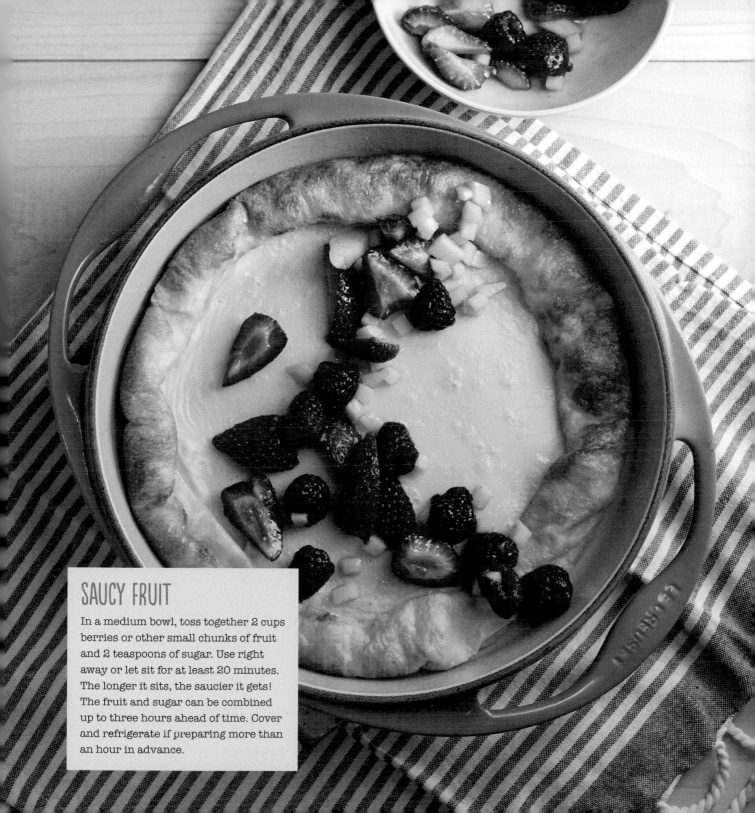

SAUCY FRUIT

In a medium bowl, toss together 2 cups berries or other small chunks of fruit and 2 teaspoons of sugar. Use right away or let sit for at least 20 minutes. The longer it sits, the saucier it gets! The fruit and sugar can be combined up to three hours ahead of time. Cover and refrigerate if preparing more than an hour in advance.

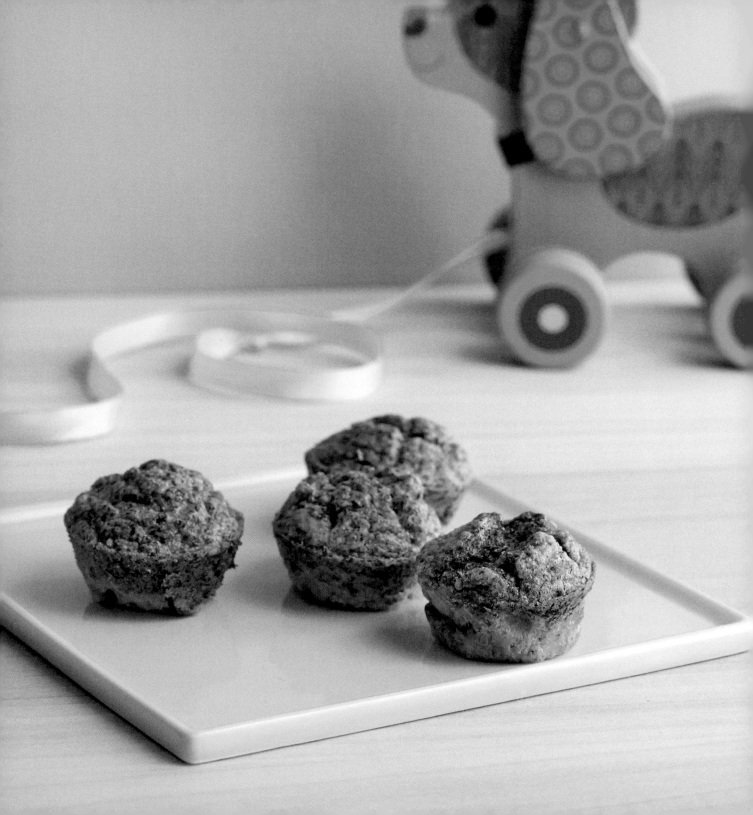

GREEN EGGS *and* BACON

Each of these toddler-sized bites has a bit of bacon and a lot of spinach inside. Make a habit of keeping frozen spinach on hand; it's a convenient way to add extra nutrition to all sorts of food, from meatballs to pasta dishes.

1 Cook the bacon in a skillet, the microwave, or a 375°F oven until just crisp. Drain on paper towels and chop into small pieces.

2 Preheat the oven to 375°F (if it isn't already). Spray a 12-cup mini muffin tin with nonstick cooking spray. Divide the chopped bacon evenly between the muffin cups.

3 In a blender, blend the spinach, eggs, and salt until smooth. Divide evenly among the bacon-filled muffin cups. Bake until the eggs are puffed and set, about 12 minutes. Let cool for 5 minutes and then remove from the muffin tin to cool on a wire rack. Serve warm or at room temperature.

Makes about 4 servings

MAKE AHEAD: Refrigerate for up to three days and reheat in the microwave or oven.

3 SLICES BACON

NONSTICK COOKING SPRAY

½ CUP FROZEN CHOPPED SPINACH, DEFROSTED AND WELL-DRAINED

4 EGGS

⅛ TEASPOON SALT

WHOLESOME TIP

Check the ingredient label for bacon made without added nitrates or nitrites, which have been linked to colon cancer.

Nutrition per serving (3 muffins): 109 calories; 8g protein; 8g fat (2g sat. fat); 2g carbohydrates; 1g fiber; 0g sugars; 284mg sodium; 50mg calcium; 1mg iron; 160mg potassium; 1mg Vitamin C; 2528IU Vitamin A

ZUCCHINI and CARROT DONUTS ❄

NONSTICK COOKING SPRAY

3 EGGS

1 CUP CANOLA OIL

¾ CUP SUGAR

1 TABLESPOON VANILLA EXTRACT

1¼ CUPS ALL-PURPOSE FLOUR

1 CUP WHOLE-WHEAT FLOUR

1 TEASPOON BAKING SODA

1 TABLESPOON CINNAMON

¾ TEASPOON NUTMEG

1 TEASPOON SALT

2 CUPS GRATED ZUCCHINI (ABOUT 1 MEDIUM)

½ CUP GRATED CARROT

Lightly spiced and just slightly sweet, these beauties are a great way to get some vegetables on the table in the morning. I love to bake them in donut tins, but they could just as easily be muffins. In fact, I often bake up a combination to avoid washing and refilling my donut tins after the first batch. Spelt flour would be a tasty replacement for the whole wheat.

1 Preheat the oven to 350°F. Spray 24 donut molds or muffin cups (or a combination) with nonstick cooking spray.

2 In a large bowl, whisk together the eggs, canola oil, sugar, and vanilla. Add the two flours, baking soda, cinnamon, nutmeg, and salt. Stir to combine. Stir in the zucchini and carrot.

3 Divide the batter evenly among the donut molds and/or muffin cups. Bake until a toothpick inserted into the center of a donut comes out with only a few crumbs clinging to it, 15 to 18 minutes (or about 5 minutes longer for muffins). Let cool for 5 minutes in the tin, then carefully remove the donuts to a rack to cool. Serve warm or at room temperature.

Makes 24 donuts or muffins

MAKE AHEAD: Store at room temperature in an airtight container for up to two days. To freeze, wrap individual muffins in foil and freeze in a zip-top bag for up to three months.

Nutrition per donut: 156 calories; 2g protein; 10g fat (1g sat. fat); 15g carbohydrates; 1g fiber; 7g sugars; 160mg sodium; 10mg calcium; 0mg iron; 62mg potassium; 2mg Vitamin C; 430IU Vitamin A

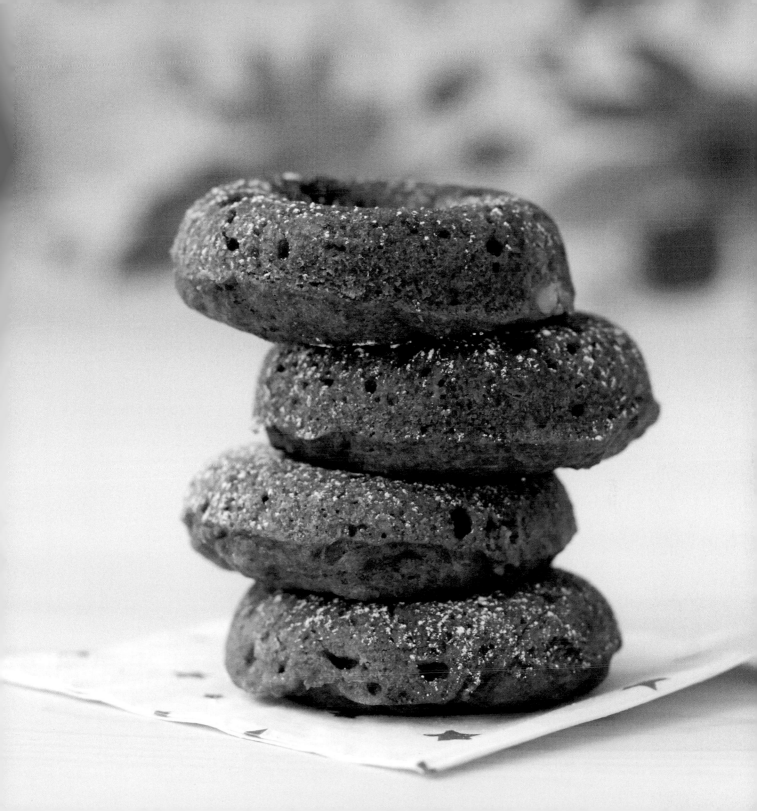

TENDER BANANA MUFFINS

4 TABLESPOONS UNSALTED
BUTTER, MELTED AND
COOLED SLIGHTLY

2 EGGS

1 TEASPOON VANILLA

¼ CUP PACKED DARK
BROWN SUGAR

¼ CUP ALL-PURPOSE FLOUR

¼ CUP SPELT OR WHOLE-
WHEAT FLOUR

2 TEASPOONS BAKING
POWDER

¼ TEASPOON SALT

1 CUP MASHED BANANA
(ABOUT 2–3 BANANAS)

These small muffins are super moist and delicious with a smear of peanut or almond butter. Be sure to use ripe, or even overripe, bananas in this recipe for maximum flavor and tenderness.

1 Preheat the oven to 350°F. Line a standard-sized muffin tin with paper liners or spray with nonstick cooking spray.

2 In a large bowl, whisk together the butter, eggs, vanilla, and brown sugar. Add the two flours, baking powder, and salt, and stir to combine. Stir in the mashed banana.

3 Divide the batter evenly among the prepared muffin cups. Bake for 15 minutes or until a toothpick inserted into the center of a muffin comes out with only a few crumbs clinging to it. Let cool for 5 minutes in the muffin tin, then carefully remove the muffins to a rack to cool. Serve warm or at room temperature.

WHOLESOME TIP

Spelt—a whole-grain variety of wheat—has a nutty sweetness perfect in baked goods. High in fiber and a good source of iron, spelt flour can be found in well-stocked grocery stores. Look for brands like Bob's Red Mill.

Makes 12 muffins

MAKE AHEAD: Store at room temperature in an airtight container for up to two days— these muffins stay tender and moist longer than many. To freeze, wrap individual muffins in foil and freeze in a zip-top bag for up to three months.

Nutrition per muffin: 97 calories; 2g protein; 5g fat (3g sat. fat); 13g carbohydrates; 1g fiber; 7g sugars; 122mg sodium; 68mg calcium; 0mg iron; 97mg potassium; 2mg Vitamin C; 170IU Vitamin A

LEEK-Y FRITTATA BITES

Frittatas may be Italy's gift to busy parents. They are delicious served warm, at room temperature, or cold. They are almost endlessly customizable. (No leeks? Sauté sliced onion. Mushrooms aren't a favorite? Use virtually any cooked veggie.) And they perform just as brilliantly for lunch or dinner. Grazie Italia!

1 Preheat the oven to 350°F.

2 Heat 1 tablespoon olive oil in a medium nonstick, oven-safe skillet, such as cast iron. Add the mushrooms and cook for 5 minutes or until golden brown. Transfer to a small bowl.

3 Add the remaining tablespoon olive oil to the skillet and reduce the heat to medium-low. Add the leeks and sauté until soft, about 10 minutes. Return the mushrooms to the pan.

4 Whisk together the eggs, salt, and pepper in a medium bowl. Pour over the leeks and mushrooms. Sprinkle with the goat cheese. Cook for 2 minutes and then transfer to the oven.

5 Bake until lightly golden and set in the middle, 12 to 15 minutes. Let sit for 5 minutes, then transfer to a plate. Slice into wedges or cut into cubes and serve.

Makes about 8 servings

MAKE AHEAD: Refrigerate for up to three days and reheat in the microwave or oven. The frittata can also be served cold or at room temperature.

Nutrition per serving: 122 calories; 7g protein; 9g fat (3g sat. fat); 4g carbohydrates; 1g fiber; 1g sugars; 231mg sodium; 50mg calcium; 1mg iron; 151mg potassium; 3mg Vitamin C; 660IU Vitamin A

2 TABLESPOONS OLIVE OIL, DIVIDED

4 OZ. CREMINI MUSHROOMS, STEMMED AND THINLY SLICED

2 MEDIUM LEEKS, WHITE AND LIGHT GREEN PARTS ONLY, HALVED LENGTHWISE AND THINLY SLICED

8 EGGS

½ TEASPOON SALT

FRESHLY GROUND PEPPER, TO TASTE

2 TABLESPOONS CRUMBLED GOAT CHEESE

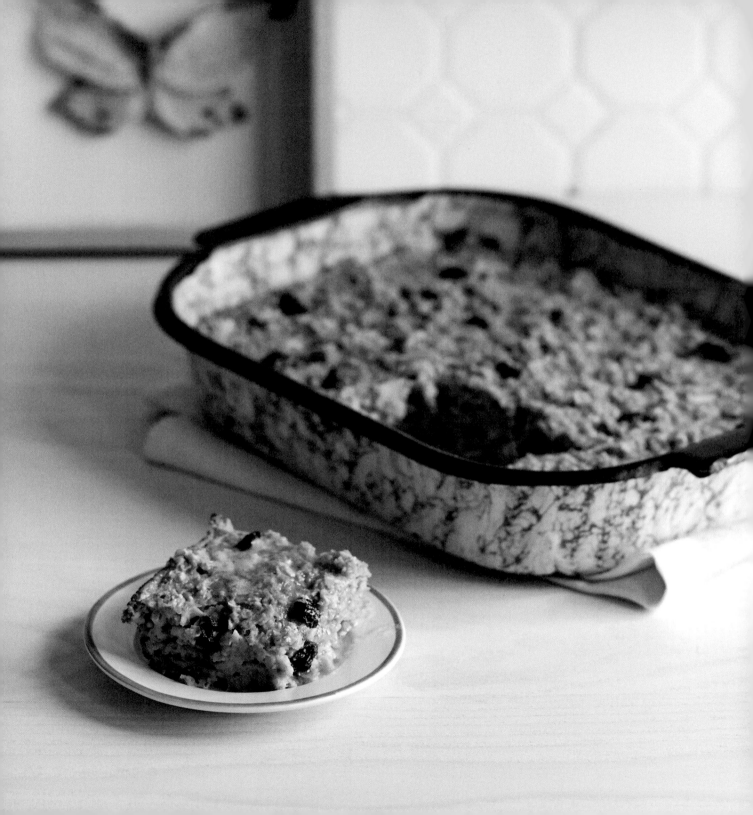

Apple-Cinnamon
BAKED OATMEAL

Searching for a wholesome weekend breakfast or brunch dish that the entire family will enjoy? Look no further than this dish inspired by Heidi Swanson. The shredded apples virtually melt into the oatmeal. And there's no need to peel them: just core and grate on a box grater or in the food processor.

1 Preheat the oven to 400°F. Butter the bottom and sides of an 8 x 8-inch baking dish.

2 In a large bowl, whisk together 1 tablespoon of the melted butter, the milk, maple syrup, egg, and vanilla. Add the oats, cinnamon, baking powder, and salt, and stir until combined; the mixture will be very milky. Stir in the grated apple and raisins.

3 Pour the oat mixture into the prepared baking dish, and press down with your hands or a spoon so all of the oats are submerged. Bake until golden brown and set in the middle, about 40 minutes. Let cool for 5 minutes. Drizzle with the remaining tablespoon of melted butter, cut into squares, and serve.

Makes about 9 servings

MAKE AHEAD: Refrigerate for up to three days and reheat in the microwave or oven. Truthfully, I also like leftovers cold with a splash of coconut milk and maple syrup.

2 TABLESPOONS UNSALTED BUTTER, MELTED AND SLIGHTLY COOLED, PLUS MORE FOR THE BAKING DISH

2 CUPS MILK

2 TABLESPOONS MAPLE SYRUP

1 EGG

1 TABLESPOON VANILLA EXTRACT

2 CUPS ROLLED OATS

1½ TEASPOONS CINNAMON

1 TEASPOON BAKING POWDER

¼ TEASPOON SALT

2½ CUPS GRATED APPLE (ABOUT 2 MEDIUM)

½ CUP RAISINS

Nutrition per serving: 210 calories; 6g protein; 6g fat (3g sat. fat); 34g carbohydrates; 4g fiber; 13g sugars; 147mg sodium; 135mg calcium; 2mg iron; 213mg potassium; 3mg Vitamin C; 225IU Vitamin A

Sugar, Sugar Everywhere...

Have you ever picked up a carton of yogurt or a package of cereal and done a double take when reading the nutrition label? These supposedly nutritious foods can contain up to 25 grams of sugar—over six teaspoons—per serving. In today's packaged food world it pays to be savvy about sugar, especially where our kids are concerned.

Sugar in our kids' diets can come in two forms: naturally occurring sugars, found in fruits, some vegetables, and dairy, and added sugars. Happily, naturally occurring sugars are A-OK since they come with vitamins, minerals, nutrients, and fiber. Fiber helps to slow down the release of sugar into the bloodstream. And, sugar in fruit is much less concentrated, so you would have to eat a lot of blueberries, for example, to get the same amount you would get in a cookie. Added sugars are the ones to try to steer clear of, except for the occasional treat.

Where can added sugars be found? Over half of the food products marketed to toddlers derive more than 20 percent of their calories from added sugar. Apart from the obvious offenders like soda, ice cream, cookies, and candy, a lot of sugar is hidden in seemingly healthier foods like flavored yogurts, granola bars, muffins, breakfast cereals, and instant oatmeal. A typical flavored yogurt may contain between two to three teaspoons, or more, of added sugar per six-ounce tub. Many granola bars have the same amount of sugar as cookies. A typical store-bought muffin brings around seven teaspoons of sugar to the table. Breakfast cereals come dusted with two to three teaspoons of sugar per serving, and instant oatmeal can add three to four teaspoons of sugar to your child's diet. When you consider that the American Heart Association recommends a maximum of 4 teaspoons of added sugar a day for kids who eat 1,200 calories (a typical daily toddler intake), it's easy to see how quickly children can eat more sugar than is healthy.

Sugar is sugar is sugar. To find out whether or not the product you are buying contains added sugar, carefully read the ingredients list. Everything ending with an "ose," like maltose or sucrose, is an added sugar, as are other ingredients like high-fructose corn syrup, molasses, cane sugar, corn sweetener, raw sugar, syrup, honey, maple syrup, and fruit juice concentrate.

So what can parents do to nip their toddler's sugar habit in the bud? First, buy unsweetened foods whenever possible and sweeten them yourself; you will invariably use less sugar than processed food manufacturers. Add honey, maple, or agave nectar to plain yogurt or oatmeal or sweeten with chopped or puréed fruit. Instead of using sugary jelly in a PB & J, slice up a banana.

And, be mindful of fruit juice, since even 100 percent juice drinks do not provide much, if any, fiber and have a high concentration of naturally occurring fruit sugar. That's why the American Academy of Pediatrics recommends avoiding fruit juice for babies under six months of age and limiting it to four to six ounces of 100 percent fruit juice for children between one and six years of age.

All that said, a small amount of sugar is actually beneficial for small children as it provides a very concentrated form of energy. So an occasional piece of cake, candy, or a cookie can be a part of a balanced diet. Just make sure treats don't become a daily occurrence and that the "healthy" foods you serve are just that.

- Natalia Stasenko, MS, RD

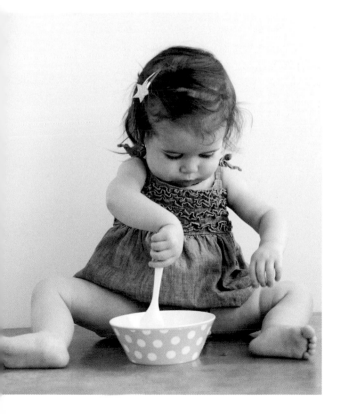

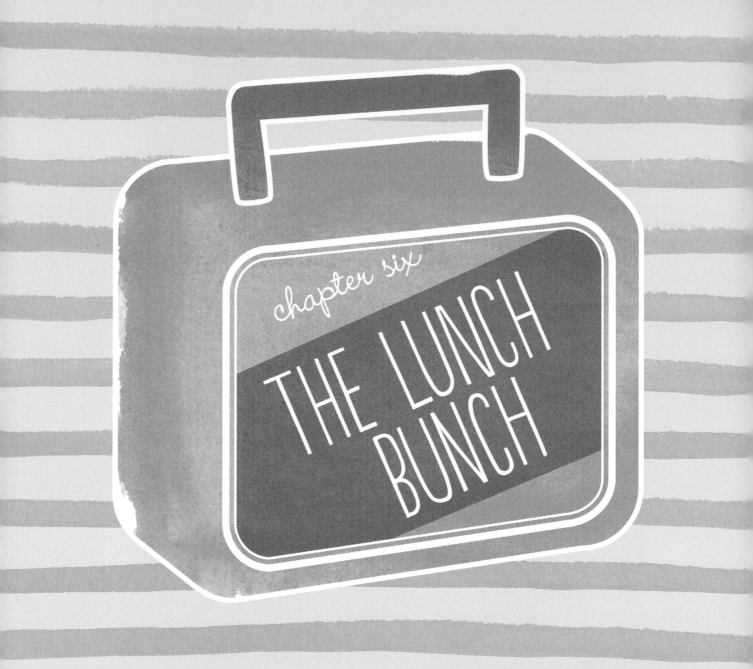

chapter six

THE LUNCH
BUNCH

MIDDAY MEALS FOR HUNGRY KIDS
(12 months and up)

At first, feeding my toddler lunch flummoxed me. I had just given Rosa a healthy breakfast, and I was already thinking ahead to our nutritious, appealing family dinner. I had to make lunch, too?

I could see how tempting it was to fall back on a daily menu of peanut butter and jelly sandwiches or frozen chicken nuggets. But since I had vowed to provide variety and home-cooked meals to my daughter whenever possible, I knew I needed to get creative.

So I made a few rules. First, with very few exceptions, lunch shouldn't take more than 20 minutes of active time to put together. Second, I would use leftovers whenever possible. Third, I would take advantage of carefully chosen pantry items so I would always have ingredients for a healthy lunch on hand.

Once I had this framework in place, lunch was no longer a burden, but instead a cornerstone of our day I could look forward to.

Each recipe in this chapter makes at least two servings: one for your toddler and one for you.

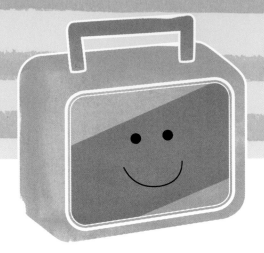

lunch made easy

As I learned when Rosa was small, convenience is the key to a healthy lunch, so don't throw away those leftovers! Get a head start (and be kind to your budget) by drawing on food that is already cooked. Even small amounts of these foods can help you get a healthy lunch on the table fast:

- Cooked chicken
- Cooked quinoa
- Cooked brown rice
- Cooked whole-grain pasta
- Vegetables purées, especially butternut squash and cauliflower
- Steamed or roasted vegetables

Also, consider going vegetarian at lunch on a regular basis—your meals will likely be faster and more budget-friendly. So while you'll see some meat in these recipes (and plenty of cheese and eggs), most of the dishes are plant-based: good for your wallet, good for your health, and good for your schedule.

On the nutrition front, strive for balance and variety at lunchtime. Each meal should include protein, fruits and/or vegetables (preferably some of both), and a healthy starch. Round out any of the recipes in this chapter with simple cut-up fruit, whole-grain crackers, or lightly steamed veggies. To drink, continue offering your child water out of an open cup.

SERVING SIZES

Each recipe in this chapter makes at least two servings—one for your toddler and one for you. The servings are more on the "adult" end of the spectrum, so don't be surprised if your toddler doesn't eat her whole portion. Leftovers for tomorrow!

TORTELLINI SOUP

In my experience tortellini soup is like catnip for toddlers (and bigger kids). Having a well-stocked pantry makes this dish come together in a snap. Frozen vegetables are a convenient substitute for the broccoli; just adjust the cooking time according to the package directions. I prefer dried tortellini to fresh or frozen for their petite size. Look for them in the pasta aisle.

1 In a medium saucepan, bring the broth to a boil. Add the tortellini and cook for 5 minutes.

2 Add the broccoli and cook for 5 minutes more or until the tortellini and the broccoli are tender. Add the salt and lemon juice. Pour into 2 serving bowls and garnish with pepper and Parmesan to taste.

Makes 2 servings

3 CUPS LOW-SODIUM CHICKEN BROTH

4 OZ. DRIED CHEESE-FILLED TORTELLINI

2 CUPS SMALL BROCCOLI FLORETS (ABOUT ½ BUNCH)

⅛ TEASPOON SALT

½ TEASPOON LEMON JUICE

FRESHLY GROUND PEPPER, TO TASTE

GRATED PARMESAN CHEESE (OPTIONAL)

Nutrition per serving: 270 calories; 19g protein; 6g fat (3g sat. fat); 38g carbohydrates; 5g fiber; 3g sugars; 617mg sodium; 146mg calcium; 2mg iron; 557mg potassium; 56mg Vitamin C; 1476IU Vitamin A

20-MINUTE MAC 'N' CHEESE

SALT

2 CUPS MULTI-GRAIN ELBOW MACARONI (8 OZ.)

2 TABLESPOONS UNSALTED BUTTER

2 TABLESPOONS FLOUR

1½ CUPS MILK

½ TEASPOON DIJON MUSTARD

1½ CUPS SHREDDED SHARP CHEDDAR CHEESE (4 OZ.)

FRESHLY GROUND PEPPER, TO TASTE

Homemade macaroni and cheese in under half an hour? You bet. This creamy mac is better tasting than any that comes from a box and better for you. (Just have a look at the ingredient list on that box.)

1 Bring a medium pot of salted water to a boil. Cook the macaroni according to package directions. Drain and return to the pot.

2 Meanwhile, melt the butter in a small saucepan over medium heat. Add the flour and whisk until smooth and bubbly. Cook for 2 minutes or until the mixture is a light tan.

3 Whisk in the milk. Bring to a simmer, whisking frequently to remove any lumps. Whisk in the mustard and ½ teaspoon salt. Simmer for 5 minutes, stirring occasionally. Remove the sauce from the heat and stir in the cheese until fully melted.

4 Pour the cheese sauce over the pasta. Stir to combine, and add freshly ground pepper to taste.

Makes about 5 servings

MAKE AHEAD: Refrigerate for up to three days. Reheat in the microwave. Or, for a crispier version, butter a baking dish, pour in the macaroni and cheese, and bake at 350°F until the top is golden brown, about 15 to 20 minutes.

Nutrition per serving: 382 calories; 17g protein; 18g fat (11g sat. fat); 38g carbohydrates; 1g fiber; 1g sugars; 483mg sodium; 346mg calcium; 2mg iron; 246mg potassium; 1mg Vitamin C; 633IU Vitamin A

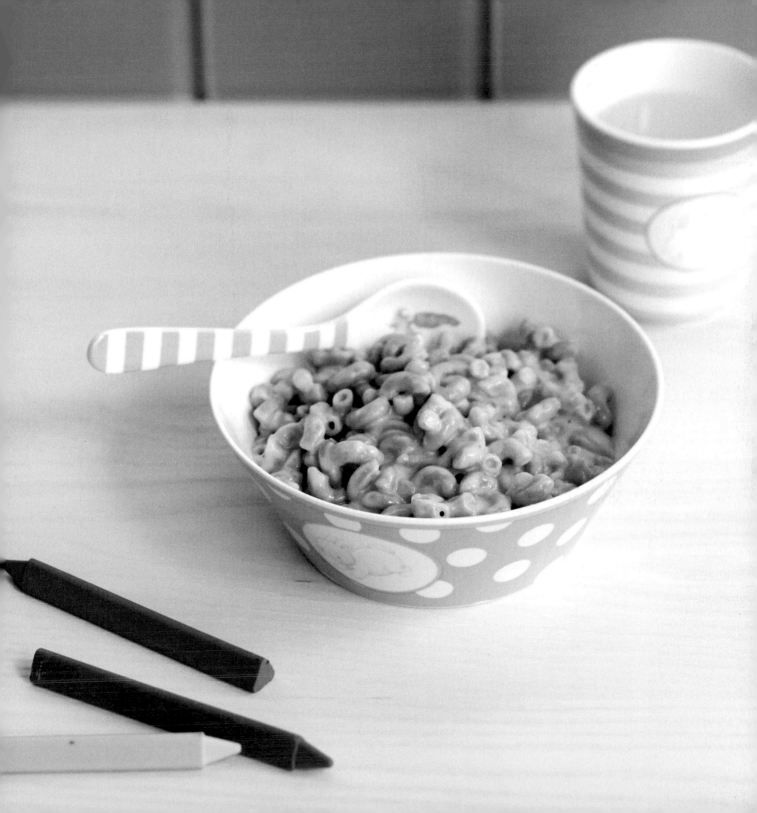

COCONUT LENTIL STEW

1 TABLESPOON PLUS 1
TEASPOON COCONUT OIL

½ CUP FINELY CHOPPED
YELLOW ONION

1 TEASPOON CUMIN

½ TEASPOON GROUND
CORIANDER

½ TEASPOON TURMERIC

3 CUPS LOW-SODIUM
CHICKEN BROTH

1 CUP RED LENTILS, RINSED

½ TEASPOON SALT, OR MORE
TO TASTE

Unsalted butter is a tasty substitute for coconut oil in this satisfying dish.

1 Heat 1 tablespoon of coconut oil in a medium saucepan over medium-low heat. Add the onion and sauté until lightly browned, 8 to 10 minutes.

2 Add the cumin, coriander, and turmeric. Stir to coat the onion and cook for 2 minutes.

3 Add the chicken broth and bring to a boil. Add the lentils and salt. Reduce the heat to medium-low, partially cover, and simmer until the lentils are tender, about 20 minutes. The lentils should be thick, not soupy. If you find that they are becoming too thick, cover the pan for the final minutes of cooking.

Makes about 3 servings

MAKE AHEAD: Store for up to three days in the refrigerator. Reheat in the microwave or on the stovetop.

Nutrition per serving: 321 calories; 21g protein; 9g fat (6g sat. fat); 43g carbohydrates; 7g fiber; 1g sugars; 465mg sodium; 42mg calcium; 5mg iron; 615mg potassium; 3mg Vitamin C; 38IU Vitamin A

STUFFED SWEET POTATOES

Yes, this recipe takes longer than 20 minutes, but only 10 minutes is active time. If you're in a rush, prick the sweet potatoes with a fork and cook in the microwave on high for six to eight minutes. You'll miss out on some of the sweet caramelization that comes from roasting, but there's no shame in a shortcut.

1 Preheat the oven to 425°F. Line a rimmed baking sheet with parchment paper or aluminum foil. Place the sweet potatoes on the baking sheet and roast until completely tender, about 35 minutes. Let cool for 5 to 10 minutes.

2 In a small microwave-safe bowl, stir together the beans and salsa. Heat in the microwave for 15 seconds.

3 Slice open the top of the sweet potatoes and open them up so they are mostly flat. Serve at the table with the cheese, bean and salsa mixture, and more salsa for topping.

Makes 2 servings

2 MEDIUM SWEET POTATOES (ABOUT 1 POUND)

½ CUP CANNED PINTO BEANS, DRAINED AND RINSED

2 TEASPOONS MILD SALSA, PLUS MORE FOR TOPPING

¼ CUP SHREDDED CHEDDAR CHEESE

Nutrition per serving (1 sweet potato with toppings): 210 calories; 9g protein; 5g fat (3g sat. fat); 33g carbohydrates; 4g fiber; 8g sugars; 254mg sodium; 174mg calcium; 2mg iron; 672mg potassium; 23mg Vitamin C; 22067IU Vitamin A

E.A.T. SANDWICH

4 SLICES WHOLE-WHEAT
BREAD, TOASTED

½ AVOCADO, MASHED

SALT

2 TEASPOONS OLIVE OIL

2 EGGS

FRESHLY GROUND PEPPER,
TO TASTE

2 SLICES TOMATO

My daughter and I love good BLTs as much as the next gals, but the E.A.T.—egg, avocado, tomato—is just as delicious and even healthier. This sandwich is especially good when tomatoes are in season. Since the ingredients in this sandwich are so simple, be sure to season it well with salt.

1 Using a 3-inch round cookie cutter, cut a large circle out of each piece of toast. Divide the mashed avocado evenly between 2 circles. Sprinkle with salt.

2 Heat the olive oil in a medium skillet over medium heat. Crack the eggs into the skillet and sprinkle with salt and pepper. Cover the pan and cook until the yolks are mostly cooked through, about 3 minutes. Flip the eggs with a spatula and remove the pan from the heat. Transfer the eggs to a cutting board and use the cookie cutter to shape them into circles. Place an egg circle on each slice of avocado-smeared toast.

3 Top the eggs with the tomato slices. Sprinkle with salt and cover with the remaining toast circles.

Makes 2 sandwiches

Nutrition per serving (1 sandwich): 442 calories; 15g protein; 21g fat (4g sat. fat); 53g carbohydrates; 9g fiber; 5g sugars; 385mg sodium; 62mg calcium; 4mg iron; 640mg potassium; 8mg Vitamin C; 477IU Vitamin A

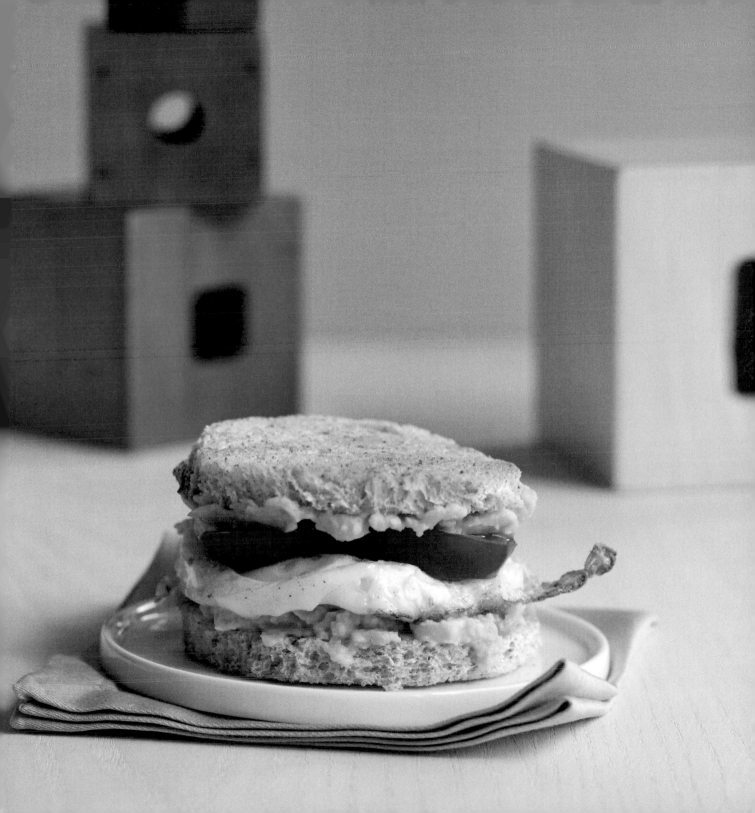

CURRIED CHICKEN SALAD *in Mini Pitas*

2 TABLESPOONS PLAIN
GREEK YOGURT

2 TABLESPOONS MAYONNAISE

1 TABLESPOON WHITE
WINE VINEGAR

1 TEASPOON CURRY POWDER

½ TEASPOON TURMERIC

½ TEASPOON SALT

1 COOKED CHICKEN
BREAST, SHREDDED (ABOUT
1¼ CUPS MEAT)

¼ CUP FINELY CHOPPED
CELERY

3 TABLESPOONS RAISINS

2 TABLESPOONS CHOPPED
CILANTRO

3 MINI PITAS, TOP ½-INCH
CUT OFF

Take advantage of leftover chicken for this recipe if you have it. But if you don't, poaching a chicken breast takes little time: simmer it in barely boiling water for about 15 minutes or until cooked through.

1 In a medium bowl, stir together the yogurt, mayonnaise, vinegar, curry powder, turmeric, and salt. Add the chicken breast, celery, and raisins and toss to coat. Stir in the cilantro.

2 Divide the chicken between the pitas and serve.

Makes 3 sandwiches

MAKE AHEAD: Chicken salad keeps in the fridge for up to three days. Serve chilled.

WHOLESOME TIP
To shred chicken, use your fingers and simply tear off pieces along the grain. Chopping is another option.

Nutrition per serving (½ cup salad and mini pita): 283 calories; 19g protein; 12g fat (2g sat. fat); 24g carbohydrates; 2g fiber; 14g sugars; 541mg sodium; 57mg calcium; 2mg iron; 254mg potassium; 2mg Vitamin C; 119IU Vitamin A

CRISPY QUESADILLAS

I could eat a freshly cooked quesadilla any day of the week, especially when it's stuffed with these wholesome and delicious ingredients. Of course, don't hesitate to vary the filling ingredients to accommodate the leftovers in your fridge. Think shredded chicken, beef, or pork, finely chopped broccoli, or even thinly sliced apples.

1 In a small bowl, mash the beans with a fork. Stir in the yogurt. Using the back of a spoon or a knife, divide the bean mixture between the two tortillas, leaving a 1-inch border around the edges. Sprinkle each with a pinch of salt.

2 In another small bowl, stir together the butternut squash purée and the shredded cheese. Spread over one half of one tortilla on top of the beans, continuing to leave a 1-inch border. Fold the tortilla over to make a half-moon. Repeat with the second tortilla.

3 Heat the canola oil in a small skillet over medium heat. Add one quesadilla to the pan and cook until it is golden brown and the cheese is melted, about 2 minutes per side. Repeat with the second quesadilla. Cut into wedges and serve.

Makes 2 servings

½ CUP CANNED LOW-SODIUM BLACK BEANS, DRAINED AND RINSED

1 TABLESPOON PLAIN GREEK YOGURT

TWO 8-INCH FLOUR TORTILLAS

⅛ TEASPOON SALT

¼ CUP BUTTERNUT SQUASH PURÉE (SEE PAGE 40)

¼ CUP SHREDDED SHARP CHEDDAR CHEESE

2 TEASPOONS CANOLA OIL

Nutrition per serving (1 quesadilla): 325 calories; 12g protein; 13g fat (4g sat. fat); 41g carbohydrates; 7g fiber; 3g sugars; 550mg sodium; 217mg calcium; 3mg iron; 476mg potassium; 13mg Vitamin C; 6100IU Vitamin A

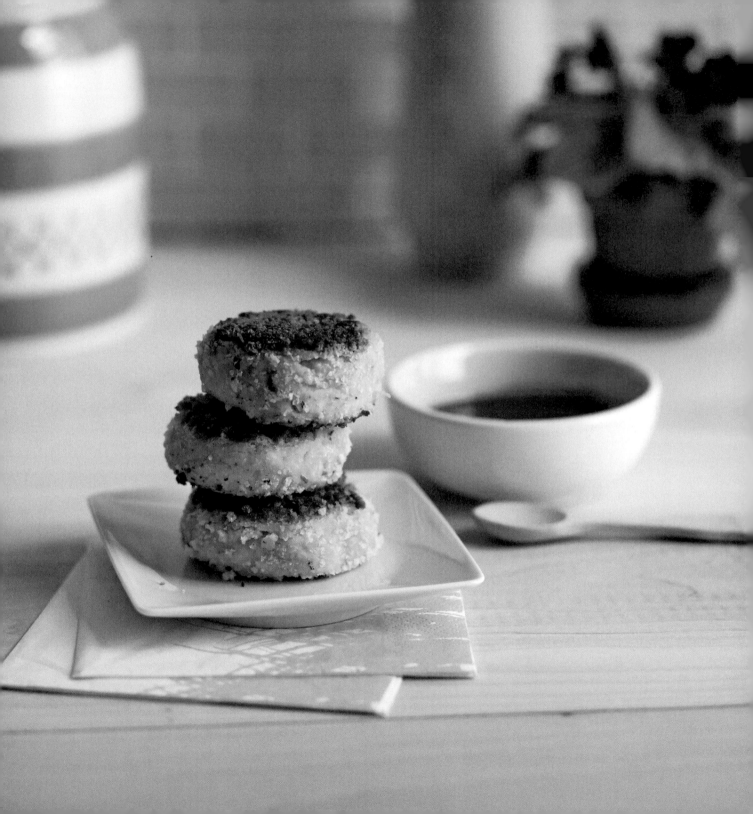

ITALIAN BEAN BURGERS

Serve these golden vegetarian patties on their own or on a bun with lettuce and tomato. They are also nice with a little Go-To Tomato Sauce (see page 191) smeared on top or set alongside as a dip.

1 In a large bowl, mash the beans with a fork or potato masher. Mix in the egg white. Add 2 tablespoons of panko, the cheese, garlic, rosemary, salt, and pepper to taste. Stir to combine. Form the bean mixture into 4 patties.

2 Heat the olive oil in a large skillet over medium-high heat. Place the remaining ⅓ cup panko in a flat dish. Dredge the patties in the panko, pressing the crumbs onto both sides and then sauté until golden, about 3 minutes per side.

Makes 4 burgers

MAKE AHEAD: Refrigerate for up to three days. You could reheat in the microwave, but the burgers will be tastier if you give them a quick sauté in olive oil.

ONE 15-OZ. CAN LOW-SODIUM CANNELLINI BEANS, DRAINED AND RINSED

1 EGG WHITE

⅓ CUP PLUS 2 TABLESPOONS PANKO

¼ CUP GRATED PARMESAN CHEESE

1 CLOVE GARLIC, FINELY CHOPPED

1 TEASPOON FINELY CHOPPED ROSEMARY

¼ TEASPOON SALT

FRESHLY GROUND PEPPER, TO TASTE

2 TABLESPOONS OLIVE OIL

Nutrition per serving (1 burger): 206 calories; 8g protein; 9g fat (2g sat. fat); 23g carbohydrates; 4g fiber; 1g sugars; 537mg sodium; 87mg calcium; 1mg iron; 41mg potassium; 0mg Vitamin C; 54IU Vitamin A

SAUSAGE-QUINOA HASH

1 FULLY COOKED CHICKEN SAUSAGE LINK, SUCH AS AIDELLS

1 TABLESPOON OLIVE OIL

1 CUP COOKED QUINOA, COLD

¼ CUP COOKED SPINACH (FROZEN AND THAWED IS FINE), LIQUID SQUEEZED OUT

½ TEASPOON SALT

FRESHLY GROUND PEPPER, TO TASTE

1 EGG, BEATEN

Use your nonstickiest pan for this flavorful—and fast—take on fried rice. A great use for leftover quinoa.

1 Cut the sausage lengthwise into quarters and slice it into bite-size pieces.

2 Heat the olive oil in a medium skillet over medium heat. Cook the sausage until browned, about 4 minutes. With a slotted spoon transfer the sausage to a bowl, leaving the fat in the pan.

3 Add the quinoa, spinach, salt, and pepper to the pan. Cook until the quinoa is lightly browned and a little crisp, about 3 minutes. Return the sausage the pan. Add the egg and stir, cooking until the egg is cooked through.

Makes 2 servings

Nutrition per serving: 272 calories; 15g protein; 14g fat (3g sat. fat); 21g carbohydrates; 3g fiber; 0g sugars; 869mg sodium; 49mg calcium; 5mg iron; 190mg potassium; 1mg Vitamin C; 173IU Vitamin A

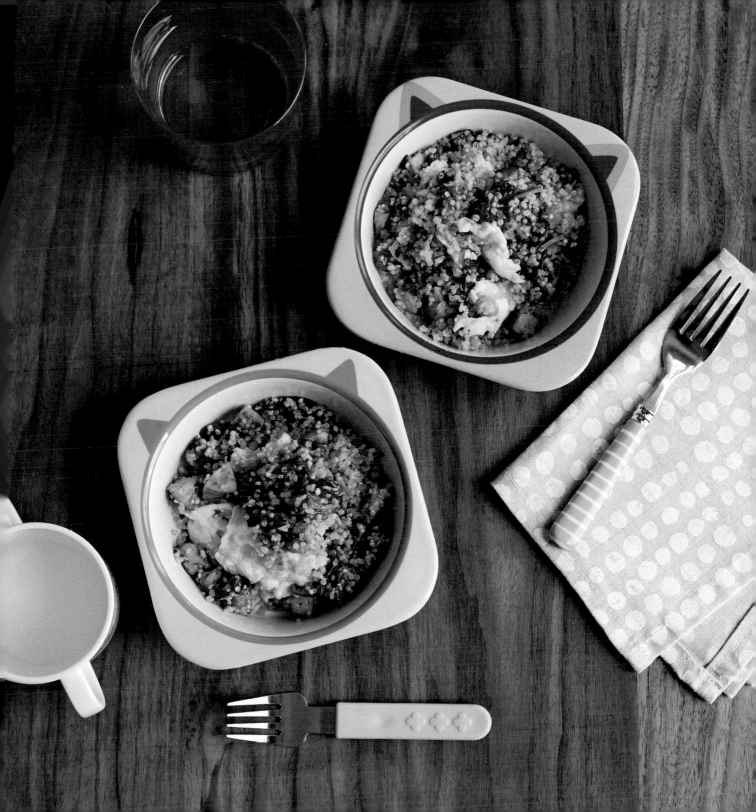

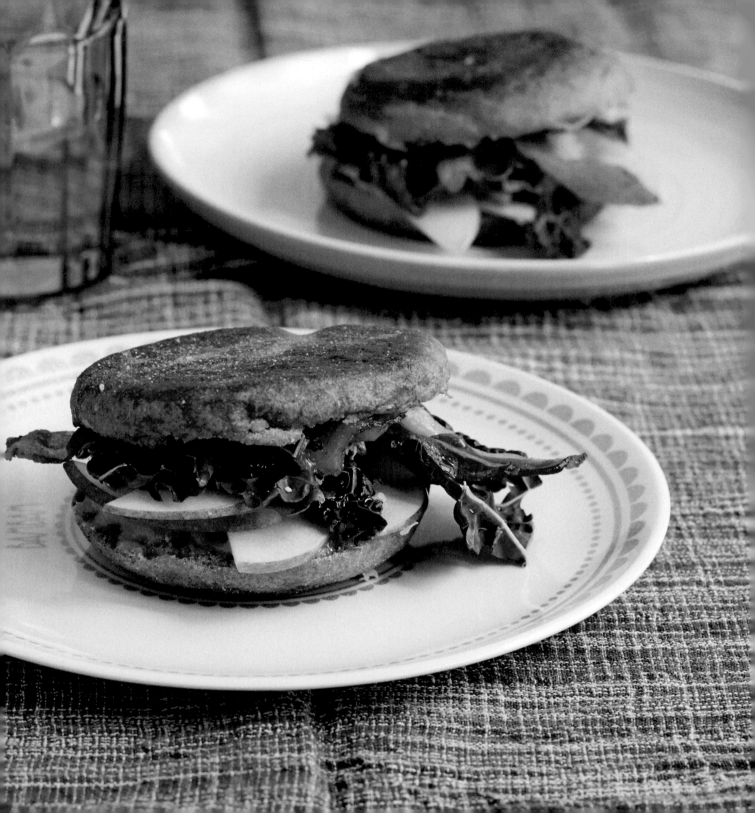

GROOVY GRILLED CHEESE

Basic grilled cheese is great, sure, but it deserves an upgrade. This version is cheesy and scrumptious (thanks, bacon!), with a pleasantly acidic bite courtesy of the apple slices. Be sure to slip in some green, whether it's a kale leaf, some spinach, or even some basil leaves. This is an opportunity to accustom your child to green in her food—it's harmless, really! Don't forget to make one of these ooey-gooey sandwiches for yourself.

2 SLICES THICK-CUT BACON

½ CUP SHREDDED SHARP CHEDDAR CHEESE

2 WHOLE-WHEAT ENGLISH MUFFINS, SPLIT AND TOASTED

2 LEAVES TUSCAN KALE, THICK STEMS REMOVED

½ SMALL APPLE, THINLY SLICED

1 Fry the bacon in a medium skillet over medium heat until just crisp. Transfer to a paper towel to drain. Pour out all but 1 teaspoon of the bacon fat.

2 Divide the shredded cheese between the bottom halves of the English muffins, reserving about 2 teaspoons. Layer the bacon, kale, apple slices, and remaining cheese. Place the tops on the English muffins.

3 Heat the pan with the bacon fat over medium heat. Add the English muffins and cook, pressing down with a spatula to flatten the sandwiches and melt the cheese. Cook until they are golden brown and the cheese is melted, 2 to 3 minutes per side.

Makes 2 sandwiches

Nutrition per serving (1 sandwich): 358 calories; 16g protein; 19g fat (9g sat. fat); 34g carbohydrates; 6g fiber; 9g sugars; 607mg sodium; 405mg calcium; 2mg iron; 325mg potassium; 22mg Vitamin C; 2887IU Vitamin A

How to Cope When Kids Get Choosy

Starting around age two, your excellent eater may start to get pickier. This is completely normal and happens for a couple of reasons. First, around this age children are growing less quickly so their bodies don't need as much energy, and they are naturally less hungry. Second, also around this time many children develop neophobia, or a fear of new foods. Scientists tell us this is a legacy of our caveman days, when tots that ran around trying any green leaf under the sun were at risk for poisoning.

While it can be frustrating to see your formerly enthusiastic eater suddenly rejecting the healthy foods she used to wolf down, take comfort in the fact that this is a normal stage. And, hopefully because you've introduced a wide variety of foods to your child during her first two years, her choosiness will be less extreme. Either way, take comfort in the fact that typically around age four children start becoming more adventurous again.

In the meantime, follow these do's and don'ts to make mealtimes as painless as possible:

Do Eat Together: Serve yourself and your child the same meal. Let him see you enjoying all the healthy foods on your plate.

Don't Force: Never pressure your child to try something or clear her plate and punish her if she doesn't. This will only make mealtimes more fraught and what should be a pleasant activity a battle. When your child is a little older you can consider making a family-wide "one polite bite" guideline, but not at this stage and only then if you are prepared to back off and carry on with the meal if your child refuses. Mealtime should never develop into a standoff at the Toddler Corral.

Do Mix It Up: At each meal be sure to serve at least one thing you know your child will eat, like whole-wheat bread, a fruit salad, or milk. But after that, don't cater the whole meal to a two-year-old's tastes. Serve a well-rounded delicious meal you'll enjoy eating. The point here is to teach your child to eat within the family structure, not to make the rest of your family eat like a toddler.

Don't Reward: Does your spouse give you a high-five when you try the sweet potato salad? No. Because it's dinner and what we do at dinner is eat. If your child tries something new don't make a big deal out of it. Also, don't promise your child a treat (food or otherwise) if she eats her meal. Then the act of eating will seem like an ordeal only to be tolerated to get to the "good stuff."

WHEN TO GET HELP

Most of the time, choosy eating in toddlers is completely normal and nothing to worry about. But on some occasions, especially if there is a concern about your child's nutrition, growth, or feeding abilities, your pediatrician may refer you to a pediatric dietitian. Here are some reasons why seeing a pediatric dietitian might be helpful for your child:

- You are worried about your child's growth and food intake.

- Your child is a very picky eater, omitting whole food groups from his diet, or has trouble tolerating certain textures, smells, or flavors.

- Your child has food allergies or sensitivities. In this case, it is important for your child's well-being to both avoid foods that may be potentially dangerous and fill the nutritional gaps that may occur in his diet.

- Your child has digestive problems.

- You have trouble introducing certain foods or textures into your baby's diet.

- Your child has a health condition such as diabetes, cerebral palsy, developmental disabilities, chronic respiratory issues, cardiac defects, or is tube fed.

The best way to find a registered dietitian who specializes in pediatrics is to ask your doctor for a referral or search the website of the Academy of Nutrition and Dietetics, www.eatright.org, for a professional in your area.

Do Deconstruct It: As often as possible give your child the chance to pick and choose what she wants to eat from what's on the table. Even the option to sprinkle on a garnish or not is empowering. Dishes in this book that can be deconstructed in full or in part are marked with the Construction Zone icon.

Don't Give Up: Your child may reject cauliflower over and over and over (and over). But don't stop serving it. Prepare it in different ways —roast it, mash it with cheese, purée it as a soup. Enjoy it yourself and eventually (it's true!) he will try it again. If you stop serving foods on his no-go list, he'll never have the chance to be adventurous when he decides he's ready.

Do Do Your Job: And then let your child do his. Your task is to provide healthy, tasty foods at mealtimes, and your child's job is to choose what and how much to eat. Period.

Do Make it Taste Good: Which would you rather eat: plain, over-boiled broccoli, or bright-green, crisp-tender broccoli drizzled with melted butter and sprinkled with salt? Guess which one your child is more likely to enjoy as well.

Don't Worry: Remember your mission as a parent is to teach your child to become a healthy eater over the long-term, not to get him to eat his pork chop on a Tuesday night.

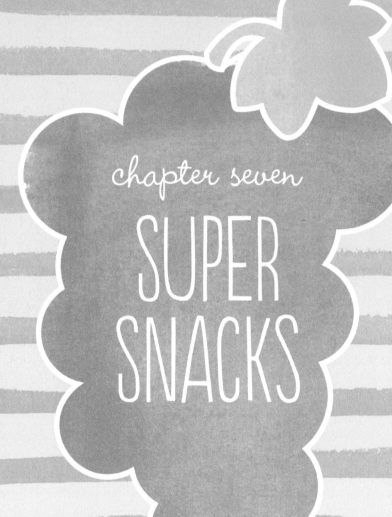

chapter seven

SUPER SNACKS

NOURISHING CHOICES FOR BETWEEN MEALS
(12 months and up)

I have a thing about snacks, so hear me out. Somehow "snacks" have become synonymous with fun, packaged foods that are more about indulgence (hence all the "guilt-free" snacks out there) than actually fulfilling dietary requirements. This isn't to say that snacks shouldn't taste good—all food should taste good! But snacks aren't extras. Thanks to their little bellies, toddlers need regular fueling with nutritious food throughout the day.

The truth is, the best snacks can be made with the foods you probably have at home already. Anything in colorful packaging, marketed to children, and even featuring "good-for-you" nutritional claims is more likely to have added sugars, salt, and fat. To top it off, chances are packaged snacks will be more expensive than the recipes in this chapter made from common nutritious staples like fruit, veggies, nuts and nut butters, whole-grain bread, and plain yogurt.

The most nutritious snacks will be well-rounded combinations of at least two food groups: whole grains, fruits/veggies, protein, and healthy fats. These heartier snacks will keep your little one satisfied longer than carbohydrate-only snacks like pretzels, crackers, and fruit.

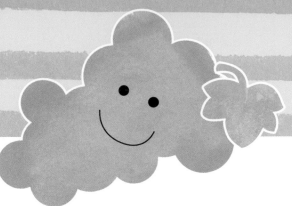

don't make this snack mistake

Snacks can be tempting for toddlers, but they're even more alluring for parents since portable snacks marketed to children make it easier than ever to always have some food on hand. Snacks seem like the perfect distraction when your little one is bored or upset, as a reward for a smooth shopping trip, or simply to entice a toddler to get in a stroller. One of the biggest favors you can do for your child's health and long-term nutritional well-being is to not make food available all day long. Using food to deal with emotions like frustration or boredom can be a hard habit to break as toddlers grow up.

Like meals, snacks should be scheduled. If they're served outside of a mealtime structure they will inevitably lead to low appetite at meals, which is when we want our kids to really eat up. To ensure a good appetite at mealtimes, plan a food-free period starting at least one and a half to two hours before a meal. During that time, serve nothing but water to your child and expect him to be comfortably hungry (but not starving) before meals.

When dinner is running a little late or your child seems to be especially hungry, offer a very light snack like a small bowl of berries, a few apple slices, or some raw vegetables. Or, if your child is not a fan of vegetables at mealtimes, try serving them as an appetizer when he is at his hungriest, while dinner finishes cooking. Try a small platter with vegetable crudités and a dip, or some cooked vegetables drizzled with olive oil and sprinkled with salt. Leftovers can be stored in the fridge and served again the next day. This little mini-snack will help your child eat better at mealtimes since being too hungry may lead to a meltdown and spoil everyone's appetite.

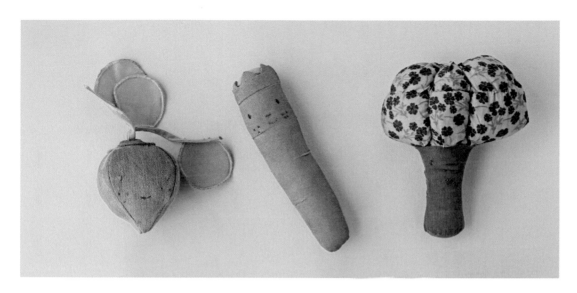

set a snack schedule

Mealtime structure becomes very important as babies switch to grown-up foods. Instead of snacking will-nilly, schedule sit-down snacks (not in the stroller or the car seat) to help set your child on a path to lifelong healthy eating.

A typical one year old will be eating three meals plus two to three snacks every day on a schedule that looks something like this:	As your child grows, they will slowly transition to eating less often. A three year old may be able to wait three to four hours between meals. His mealtime schedule may look like this:
• Milk in the morning • Breakfast • **Midmorning snack** • Lunch • **Midafternoon snack** • Dinner	• Breakfast • **Midmorning snack** • Lunch • **Midafternoon snack** • Dinner

RAINBOW KABOBS
with Lime-Yogurt Dipping Sauce

For the dip:

½ CUP PLAIN GREEK YOGURT

1½ TEASPOONS HONEY

½ TEASPOON LIME JUICE

¼ TEASPOON VANILLA EXTRACT

LIME ZEST, FOR GARNISH

For the kabobs:

A VARIETY OF COLORFUL FRUIT. MY FAVORITES, IN RAINBOW ORDER:

RASPBERRIES AND/OR STRAWBERRIES

APRICOT, PEACH, OR MANGO

PINEAPPLE

KIWI

BLUEBERRIES

BLACKBERRIES

Sweet fruit and protein-rich yogurt team up for a snack that is as colorful as it is healthy. A cocktail straw makes for a kid-safe skewer. And don't pass up the opportunity to use this simple snack as an opportunity to practice naming colors!

In a small serving bowl, stir together the yogurt, honey, lime juice, and vanilla. Sprinkle with a pinch of lime zest. Thread the fruit onto child-safe skewers and serve with the dip.

Makes 1 serving

MAKE AHEAD: Keep the yogurt dip in the fridge for up to three days. Double or triple the recipe to have extra on hand at a moment's notice.

Nutrition per serving (with ½ cup mixed fruit): 171 calories; 11g protein; 6g fat (4g sat. fat); 19g carbohydrates; 2g fiber; 17g sugars; 42mg sodium; 133mg calcium; 0mg iron; 125mg potassium; 45mg Vitamin C; 181IU Vitamin A

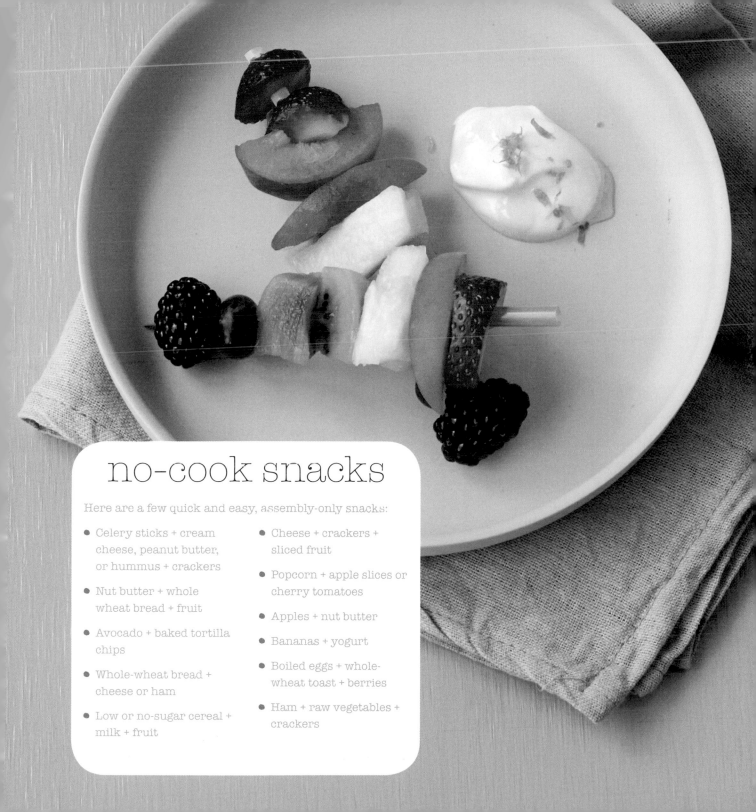

no-cook snacks

Here are a few quick and easy, assembly-only snacks:

- Celery sticks + cream cheese, peanut butter, or hummus + crackers

- Nut butter + whole wheat bread + fruit

- Avocado + baked tortilla chips

- Whole-wheat bread + cheese or ham

- Low or no-sugar cereal + milk + fruit

- Cheese + crackers + sliced fruit

- Popcorn + apple slices or cherry tomatoes

- Apples + nut butter

- Bananas + yogurt

- Boiled eggs + whole-wheat toast + berries

- Ham + raw vegetables + crackers

SMOKED TROUT _mini_ BAGELS

½ CUP CREAM CHEESE, SOFTENED

ONE 3-OZ. TIN SMOKED TROUT, DRAINED

1 TABLESPOON CHOPPED CHIVES

½ TEASPOON LEMON JUICE

PINCH SALT

FRESHLY GROUND PEPPER, TO TASTE

For serving:

1 WHOLE-WHEAT MINI BAGEL, HALVED AND TOASTED

My daughter has gone crazy for this smoked trout spread since she was three years old. We also like it spread on crackers for a hors d'oeuvre.

1 In a small bowl, mix together the cream cheese, trout, chives, lemon juice, salt, and pepper with a fork. Taste for seasoning and add more lemon, salt, or pepper if desired.

2 Spread 2 tablespoons trout spread on the mini bagel.

Makes ¾ cup spread

MAKE AHEAD: Smoked trout spread keeps well in the fridge for up to five days.

Nutrition per serving: 200 calories; 8g protein; 9g fat (4g sat. fat); 21g carbohydrates; 3g fiber; 1g sugars; 278mg sodium; 32mg calcium; 1mg iron; 27mg potassium; 0mg Vitamin C; 260IU Vitamin A

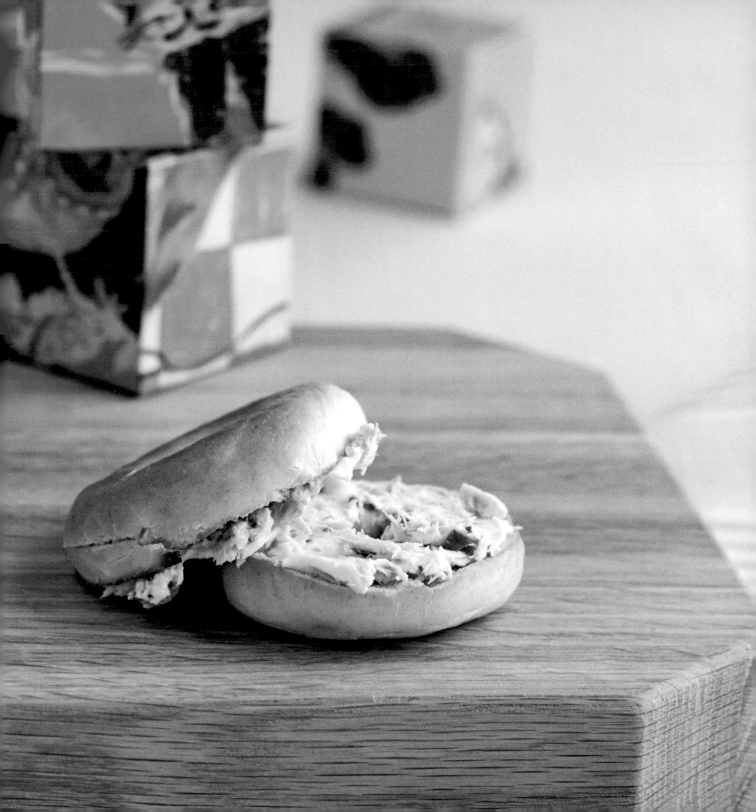

COCOA PEANUT BUTTER "ICE CREAM"

2 BANANAS, PEELED, SLICED, AND FROZEN

2 TABLESPOONS CREAMY PEANUT BUTTER

1 TEASPOON COCOA POWDER

Versions of this recipe have been zipping around the Internet faster than a toddler in a toy store. Once you taste it you'll know why.

Let the frozen bananas sit at room temperature for 5 minutes. Place in the food processor with the peanut butter and cocoa powder. Process until smooth.

Makes 2 servings

Nutrition per serving: 197 calories; 6g protein; 8g fat (2g sat. fat); 31g carbohydrates; 5g fiber; 15g sugars; 6mg sodium; 17mg calcium; 1mg iron; 436mg potassium; 10mg Vitamin C; 75IU Vitamin A

NO-BAKE SUNFLOWER DATE COOKIES

These little "cookies" are full of good stuff we want our kids to eat: nuts, seeds, and dried fruit. Even better, they only take about 15 minutes to come together. Substitute sunflower butter for the almond butter and these treats are a nut-free snack for daycares and preschools.

1   Place the raisins and vanilla in a small bowl; cover with ½ cup boiling water. Soak for about 5 minutes or until a bit plumped up. Drain.

2   Put the sunflower seeds and dates in a food processor and pulse until combined. Add the raisins, almond butter, and cinnamon. Process until smooth. It will be thick and sticky in the bowl.

3   Form the mixture into balls and flatten. If desired, top with a sprinkling of cinnamon. Refrigerate for about 2 hours or until firm.

Makes about 20 cookies

MAKE AHEAD: Keep these cookies covered in the fridge for up to a week.

1 CUP RAISINS

1 TABLESPOON VANILLA EXTRACT

½ CUP BOILING WATER

2 CUPS RAW, UNSALTED SUNFLOWER SEEDS

1 CUP DATES, PREFERABLY MEDJOOL, PITTED

2 TABLESPOONS ALMOND BUTTER

½ TEASPOON CINNAMON, PLUS MORE FOR GARNISH

Nutrition per serving (2 cookies): 176 calories; 3g protein; 7g fat (1g sat. fat); 30g carbohydrates; 3g fiber; 23g sugars; 3mg sodium; 40mg calcium; 1mg iron; 341mg potassium; 1mg Vitamin C; 33IU Vitamin A

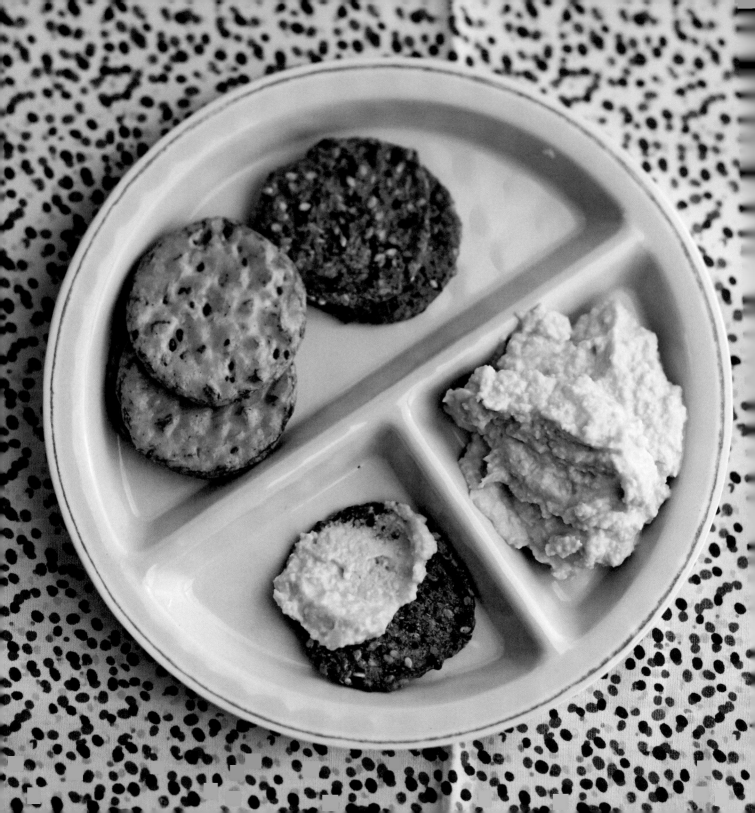

EDAMAME HUMMUS

Serve this fresh spin on hummus with whole-grain or rice crackers or veggies for dipping.

Place all of the ingredients except for the cilantro in the food processor and process until smooth. Add the cilantro and pulse until incorporated (you will still see some of the leaves).

Makes about 1 cup

MAKE AHEAD: Cover and store in the refrigerator for up to two days.

6 OZ. FROZEN SHELLED EDAMAME, DEFROSTED (ABOUT 1 CUP)

¼ CUP OLIVE OIL

¼ CUP WATER

1 TABLESPOON LIME JUICE

½ TEASPOON GRATED FRESH GINGER

¾ TEASPOON SALT

½ CUP CHOPPED CILANTRO

Nutrition per serving (2 tablespoons): 76 calories; 2g protein; 7g fat (1g sat. fat); 2g carbohydrates; 1g fiber; 0g sugars; 219mg sodium; 10mg calcium; 0mg iron; 78mg potassium; 2mg Vitamin C; 68IU Vitamin A

Banana Bread
QUINOA COOKIES

1½ CUPS WHOLE-WHEAT FLOUR

½ TEASPOON SALT

½ TEASPOON CINNAMON

½ TEASPOON BAKING POWDER

½ TEASPOON BAKING SODA

½ CUP MELTED COCONUT OIL

½ CUP PACKED BROWN SUGAR

2 LARGE EGGS

1 TEASPOON VANILLA

1 CUP COOKED QUINOA, COOLED

⅓ CUP RAW WALNUTS, VERY FINELY CHOPPED

1 BANANA, DICED

These healthy cookies (yes, healthy cookies!) are a sweet, crunchy, chewy, and satisfying snack for the whole family. They taste like decadent banana bread, but they're secretly packed with protein and fiber.

1 Preheat the oven to 375°F and line 2 rimmed baking sheets with parchment paper.

2 In a medium bowl, whisk together the flour, salt, cinnamon, baking powder, and baking soda. Set aside.

3 With an electric mixer, mix together the coconut oil and brown sugar until thoroughly combined. Add the eggs and vanilla and mix well, about 2 more minutes.

4 Add the flour mixture, mixing until just combined. Stir in the quinoa, walnuts, and banana.

5 Drop rounded tablespoonfuls of dough onto the prepared sheets an inch or so apart. Flatten each cookie slightly with your palm, and bake until lightly browned, about 12 minutes. Cool on a wire rack.

Makes about 30 cookies

MAKE AHEAD: Keep in an airtight container at room temperature for up to two days.

Nutrition per serving (1 cookie): 91 calories; 2g protein; 5g fat (3g sat. fat); 11g carbohydrates; 1g fiber; 4g sugars; 73mg sodium; 17mg calcium; 0mg iron; 63mg potassium; 0mg Vitamin C; 27IU Vitamin A

SUNNY BANANA GRAHAMS

Think of these graham cracker sandwiches as a healthier version of a s'more. For a special treat, slip in a square of chocolate or a dollop of marshmallow fluff.

In a small bowl, stir together the banana and cinnamon. Spread on 2 of the graham cracker squares. Spread the sunflower seed butter on the other 2 squares and sandwich with the banana-smeared squares.

Makes 1 serving

4 TEASPOONS MASHED BANANA

PINCH CINNAMON

2 GRAHAM CRACKERS, BROKEN INTO 4 SQUARES

1 TABLESPOON SUNFLOWER SEED BUTTER OR OTHER NUT BUTTER

Nutrition per serving: 221 calories; 6g protein; 10g fat (2g sat. fat); 28g carbohydrates; 3g fiber; 9g sugars; 190mg sodium; 32mg calcium; 2mg iron; 100mg potassium; 1mg Vitamin C; 0IU Vitamin A

HONEY-ROASTED CHICKPEAS

1 TABLESPOON OLIVE OIL

1 TABLESPOON HONEY

½ TEASPOON CINNAMON

¼ TEASPOON SALT

ONE 15-OZ. CAN LOW-SODIUM CHICKPEAS, DRAINED, RINSED, AND PATTED DRY

It's tough to stop eating roasted chickpeas, especially when they're seasoned with cinnamon and honey. This crunchy snack is also a delicious lunchbox addition or salad topper.

1 Preheat the oven to 425°F. Line a rimmed baking sheet with parchment paper.

2 In a medium-sized bowl, stir together the olive oil, honey, cinnamon, and salt. Add the chickpeas and stir to coat.

3 Spread the chickpeas onto the baking sheet and roast until crispy, about 30 minutes.

Makes 1½ cups

MAKE AHEAD: Cover in an airtight container and store at room temperature for up to two days. If you'd like, re-crisp the chickpeas in a 250°F oven for a few minutes before serving.

Nutrition per serving (¼ cup): 115 calories; 4g protein; 3g fat (0g sat. fat); 19g carbohydrates; 3g fiber; 3g sugars; 309mg sodium; 25mg calcium; 1mg iron; 124mg potassium; 3mg Vitamin C; 15IU Vitamin A

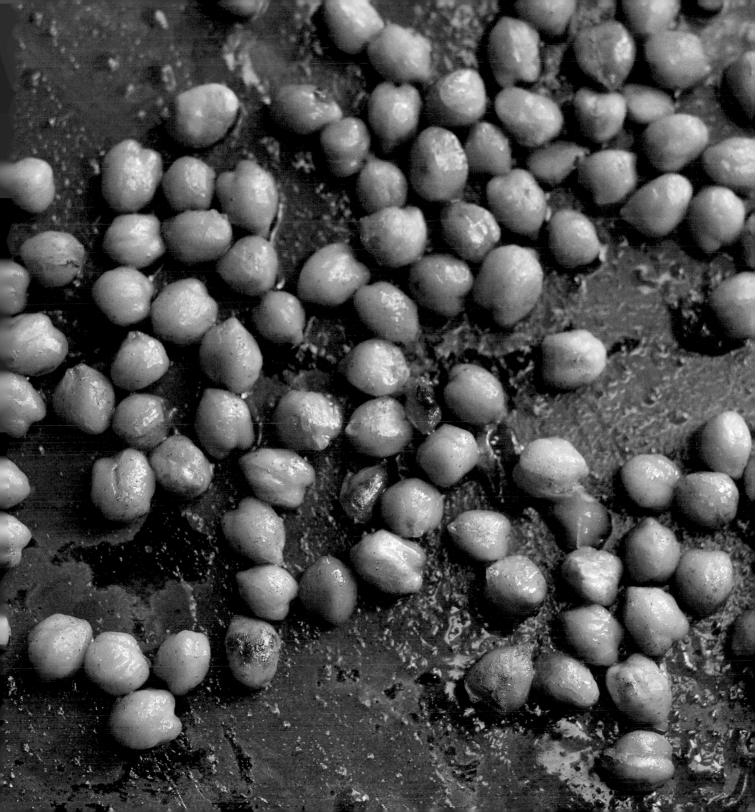

PEANUT BUTTER AND STRAWBERRY ROLL-UPS

1 TABLESPOON PEANUT BUTTER

ONE 8-INCH WHOLE-WHEAT TORTILLA

¼ CUP FINELY CHOPPED STRAWBERRIES

This snack is about as easy as they come, and a satisfying combination of protein, whole grains, and vitamin C-rich fruit. Of course, you could serve this as a roll-up, but cutting the wrap into bite-sized pieces adds an undeniable fun factor.

Spread the peanut butter on the tortilla. Add the strawberries. Roll up and slice into 1-inch thick pieces.

Makes 1 roll-up

WHOLESOME TIP

Start your toddler early on unsweetened and unsalted natural peanut butter. She'll never miss the sugar found in more processed brands.

Nutrition per serving: 247 calories; 8g protein; 11g fat (2g sat. fat); 30g carbohydrates; 4g fiber; 4g sugars; 298mg sodium; 76mg calcium; 2mg iron; 134mg potassium; 24mg Vitamin C; 5IU Vitamin A

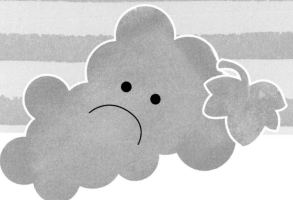

the downsides of pouches

Over the last few years pouches of fruit and/or veggie purées have become incredibly popular toddler snacks. And although there is nothing terribly wrong nutritionally with purée in pouches, and there are many delicious, additive-free and even organic options, there are three issues that experts are concerned about.

First, eating from a pouch during a formative period when oral-motor and utensil-using skills are built may slow down a child's development. Second, although many of the pouches boast a variety of vegetables like broccoli or even kale on the front label, they all taste sweet because typically the prevailing ingredient is a fruit purée or a sweet, easy-to-like vegetable like carrot. So if you would like your child to learn to enjoy kale, give him...kale, not a pouch where the flavor of kale is diluted and masked by apple or pear. Finally, since pouches are so portable, they also encourage eating outside of the mealtime structure—in the car, the stroller, or toddling around the house. This makes it easy for kids to overdo snacks and not be hungry at mealtimes.

STICKY RICE BALLS

3 CUPS WATER

2 CUPS SUSHI RICE

SALT

2 TABLESPOONS PLUS ½ TEASPOON TOASTED WHITE OR BLACK SESAME SEEDS

8 OZ. SALMON FILLET

1 TEASPOON SESAME OIL

MAKE AHEAD: Wrap individually in plastic wrap, and refrigerate for up to three days, or freeze for up to three months.

These rice balls are a riff on a popular Japanese bento box staple. If the recipe looks long, fear not. You'll be turning out rice balls in no time flat! For extra flavor, serve with the Sesame-Soy Dipping Sauce on page 206.

1 **To make the rice:** In a medium saucepan, bring the water, rice, and ½ teaspoon salt to a boil. Reduce the heat, cover, and simmer for 20 minutes, until all liquid is absorbed. Turn off the heat and let stand for 10 minutes. Stir in 2 tablespoons sesame seeds.

2 **To make the salmon:** Preheat the oven to 400°F. Line a rimmed baking sheet with parchment paper. Place the salmon on the baking sheet and rub with the sesame oil. Sprinkle with a healthy pinch of salt and ½ teaspoon sesame seeds. Bake for 15 minutes. Allow to cool, then lift the salmon off of the skin, place it in a bowl, and flake with a fork. Set aside.

3 **To assemble the rice balls:** When the rice is still hot but cool enough to handle, wet a ⅓ measuring cup. Fill the cup loosely with warm rice. Poke a hole in the middle of the rice, about halfway down. Press a scant tablespoon of salmon into the hole. Top with more rice, filling to the brim and covering the filling completely, then press down firmly to pack the cup tightly. Gently shake the rice out of the cup, and with wet hands shape the rice into a ball. Repeat with the remaining ingredients, re-wetting your hands whenever the rice gets too sticky.

Makes about 15 two-inch rice balls

Nutrition per serving (2 rice balls): 108 calories; 8g protein; 5g fat (1g sat. fat); 9g carbohydrates; 1g fiber; 0g sugars; 181mg sodium; 41mg calcium; 1g iron; 184mg potassium; 0mg Vitamin C; 13IU Vitamin A

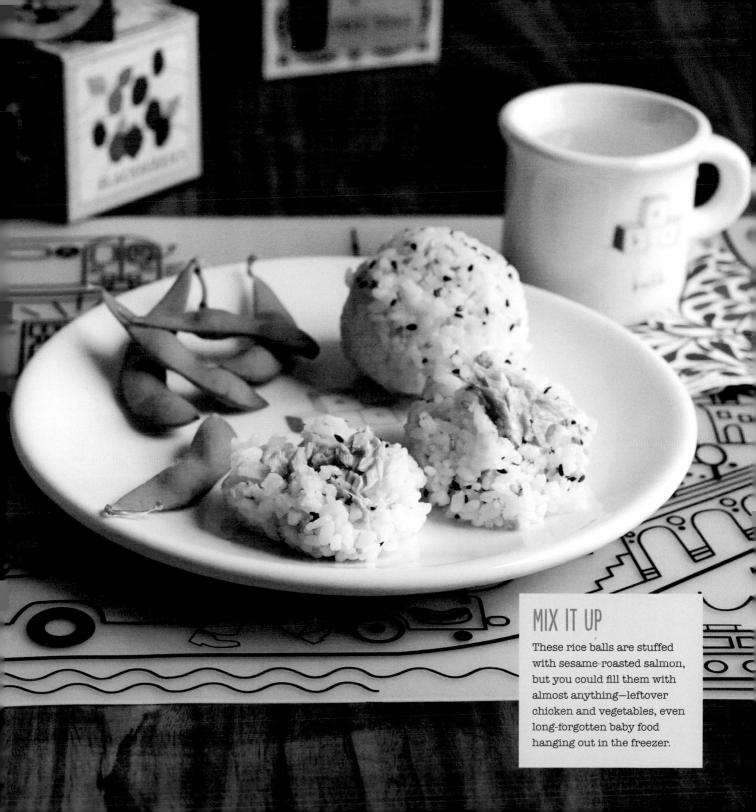

MIX IT UP

These rice balls are stuffed with sesame-roasted salmon, but you could fill them with almost anything—leftover chicken and vegetables, even long-forgotten baby food hanging out in the freezer.

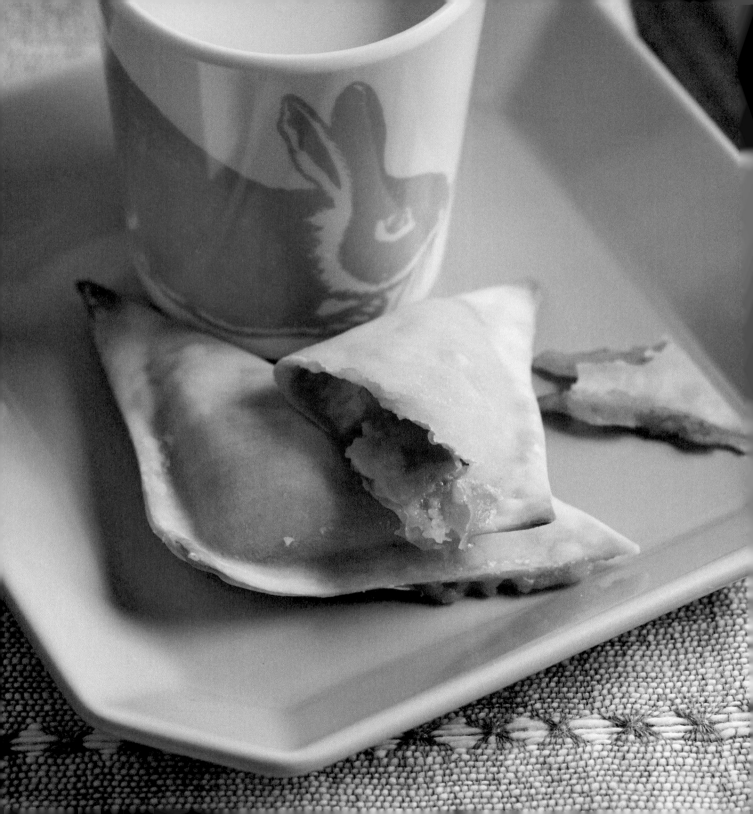

Crispy Butternut
SQUASH TRIANGLES

Wonton wrappers are a fabulous delivery mechanism for all kinds of yummy and nutritious foods. Whatever your little one's favorite food is, it probably works in a wonton wrapper. Mozzarella + sauce = pizza triangles. Spiced ground beef + mild salsa + cheese = taco triangles. Cream cheese + berries + a dusting of cinnamon/sugar = stuffed French toast triangles. Have fun!

1 Preheat the oven to 375°F. Line a rimmed baking sheet with parchment paper.

2 In medium bowl, combine the squash, cheese, onion powder, and garlic powder. Mix well. Working with one wonton wrapper at a time, top each with a teaspoon of squash and cheese filling. Using your fingertips or a pastry brush, moisten the edges with water and fold diagonally, pressing lightly to seal. Place on the prepared baking sheet. Repeat with remaining filling and wrappers.

3 Brush each triangle with oil. Bake for 12 to 15 minutes or until golden brown, turning once. Serve warm.

Makes 30 stuffed wontons

MAKE AHEAD: Refrigerate the wontons in an airtight container for up to five days. To reheat, warm in a 250°F oven for a couple of minutes. Or, freeze for up to three months. To defrost, place directly in a 350°F oven for about five to ten minutes.

1 CUP BUTTERNUT SQUASH PURÉE (SEE PAGE 40) OR CANNED PUMPKIN PURÉE

1 CUP SHREDDED CHEDDAR CHEESE

½ TEASPOON ONION POWDER

⅛ TEASPOON GARLIC POWDER

30 WONTON WRAPPERS

OLIVE OIL

Look for wonton wrappers in your grocery store's frozen section or near the tofu.

Nutrition per serving (2 wontons): 81 calories; 3g protein; 4g fat (2g sat. fat); 9g carbohydrates; 1g fiber; 0g sugars; 120mg sodium; 67mg calcium; 1mg iron; 63mg potassium; 3mg Vitamin C; 1400IU Vitamin A

CHIA PUDDING

For the pudding:

¼ CUP CHIA SEEDS

1 CUP MILK

1 TABLESPOON AGAVE NECTAR

To serve:

¼ CUP CHOPPED MANGO OR OTHER FRUIT

½ TABLESPOON SLICED ALMONDS, TOASTED

AGAVE NECTAR (OPTIONAL)

Fiber-rich chia seeds look unassuming, but they have a trick up their sleeve. Soak them in a liquid and they swell, creating a pudding-like consistency. Feel free to swap in dairy-free milk like unsweetened almond milk or coconut milk, although keep in mind that you'll lose several grams of protein.

1 In a medium-sized bowl, whisk together the chia seeds, milk, and 1 tablespoon agave nectar. Whisk well to disperse any clumped chia seeds. Cover and refrigerate at least 4 hours and preferably overnight. (If you remember, give the pudding a quick whisk an hour after you refrigerate it.)

2 To serve, top ½ cup of the chia pudding with the fruit, sliced almonds, and additional agave, if using.

Makes 2 servings

MAKE AHEAD: Store the pudding (without toppings) in the refrigerator for up to three days.

Nutrition per serving (½ cup pudding, ¼ cup fruit, and ½ tablespoon almonds): 258 calories; 11g protein; 13g fat (3g sat. fat); 31g carbohydrates; 11g fiber; 24g sugars; 62mg sodium; 285mg calcium; 2mg iron; 260mg potassium; 17mg Vitamin C; 699IU Vitamin A

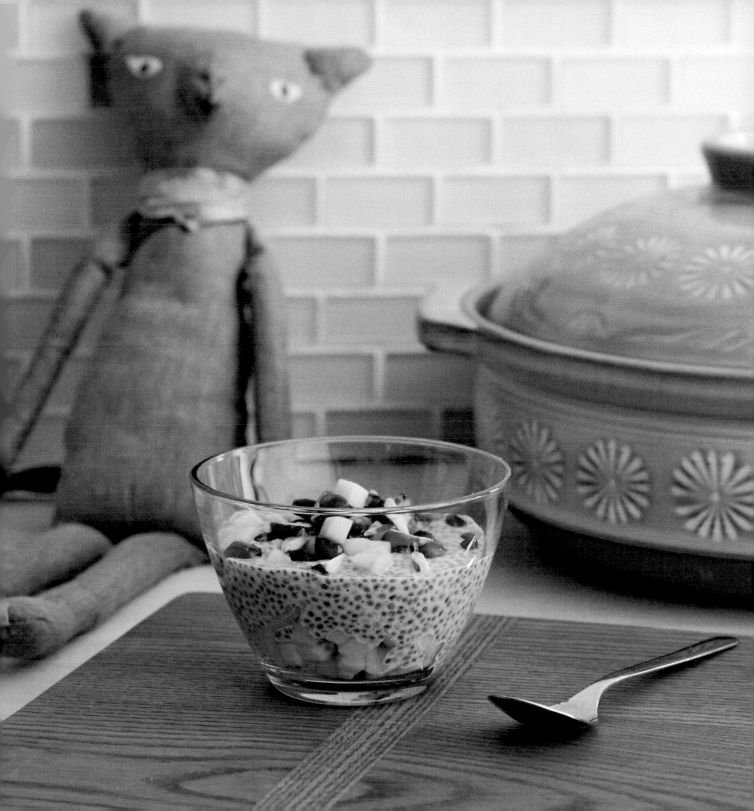

A.B.&J. *mini muffin* SANDWICHES

½ CUP WHOLE-WHEAT PASTRY FLOUR

½ CUP ALL-PURPOSE FLOUR

1½ TEASPOONS BAKING POWDER

½ TEASPOON CINNAMON

¼ TEASPOON SALT

½ CUP MILK

¼ CUP OLIVE OIL

¼ CUP PACKED DARK BROWN SUGAR

1 EGG

1 CUP SHREDDED APPLE

2 TABLESPOONS SLICED ALMONDS

For serving:

2 TEASPOONS ALMOND BUTTER

½ TEASPOON JAM

Little hands will love these sandwiches made with whole-wheat apple mini muffins. Use whole-wheat pastry flour if possible. It bakes up lighter than traditional whole wheat.

1 Preheat the oven to 375°F. Line a 24-cup mini muffin tin with paper liners or spray with nonstick cooking spray.

2 In a large bowl, whisk together the two flours, baking powder, cinnamon, and salt.

3 In a medium bowl, whisk together the milk, olive oil, dark brown sugar, and egg. Stir the wet ingredients into the dry ingredients until almost combined. Add the apple and stir until just combined.

4 Divide the batter evenly between the muffin cups. Sprinkle with the sliced almonds. Bake until a toothpick inserted in the center of a muffin comes out clean, about 14 minutes. Let cool in the pan for 5 minutes. Transfer to a wire rack and cool completely.

5 To serve, slice the tops off of 2 muffins. Spread the bottoms with almond butter and jam. Crown with the muffin tops.

Makes 24 mini muffins

MAKE-AHEAD: Keep in an airtight container at room temperature for up to two days. To freeze, wrap each mini muffin in aluminum foil and freeze in a zip-top bag. Defrost at room temperature for about an hour.

Nutrition per serving (2 muffin "sandwiches"): 199 calories; 5g protein; 12g fat (1g sat. fat); 20g carbohydrates; 2g fiber; 8g sugars; 108mg sodium; 106mg calcium; 1mg iron; 138mg potassium; 1mg Vitamin C; 50IU Vitamin A

Drink Up

Choosing the right beverages for your toddler to enjoy during and between meals and snacks can make a big difference both in his nutritional status and appetite at mealtimes.

What to offer between meals?

One word: water.

With the advent of sippy cups and juice boxes with straws, it couldn't be easier to bring juice, juice drinks, and milk with you wherever you go and watch your toddler fill up on liquids all day long. But this habit does nothing to develop good eating habits or build up an appetite for meals.

The best between-meals and snack time drink for little bodies is that oldie but goodie: water. Don't assume that children won't like plain water. If this is their go-to drink from an early age they will come to appreciate its clean, refreshing quality.

Even 100 percent fruit juice should be limited to four to six ounces a day in kids ages one to six. Too much of it on a daily basis may result in both under- and overweight children as well as iron deficiency. Although fruit juice provides some nutrition, such as good amounts of vitamin C, it lacks the fiber found in whole fruit. It also contains a higher proportion of fruit sugar per unit of weight than fruit. Think about this: In order to make a glass of orange juice, you would have to squeeze the juice from three oranges. This makes the sugar content of a glass of orange juice equal to that in three oranges, but without the beneficial fiber that slows down the release of sugar into the bloodstream and contributes to satiety. Consider approaching fruit juice and fruit juice drinks as dessert or special treat drinks in order to create more structure around their consumption.

It may seem counter-intuitive, but allowing kids to drink milk at any point throughout the day isn't a good idea either. Although more nutritious than fruit juice, milk is very easy to like for many kids, and it is very filling. An eight-ounce cup of white milk contains the same number of calories as two eggs, so if your toddler drinks three bottles or more daily, especially close to mealtimes, don't be surprised to see a lack of interest in meals, which is often interpreted as "picky eating."

Instead, approach milk as a food, not a drink, and limit its consumption to mealtimes and snacks. All dairy, including milk, should be limited to two servings a day for toddlers. One serving of dairy is eight ounces of milk or yogurt or one and a half ounces of cheese. More than that may result in lower intake of other nutritious foods and even iron deficiency since milk inhibits the absorption of iron.

Low-fat milk is not appropriate for babies and younger toddlers, but you can start making a transition to reduced-fat dairy once your child is two years old.

- Natalia Stasenko, MS, RD

chapter eight

FAMILY DINNER

TEMPTING DISHES
FOR THE WHOLE FAMILY TO SHARE
(12 months and up)

From the day I began feeding Rosa solids, I felt like I was building up to one thing: family dinner, a sometimes relaxed, sometimes rushed, occasionally frustrating, frequently enjoyable ritual we would share for years to come.

As soon as your child has moved beyond purées (if not before) try to eat together as a family as often as possible. Your child will learn so much from simply watching you use your napkin, hold a fork properly, and sample new foods with enthusiasm. Early habits are hard to break, so take this opportunity to ensure your toddler's mealtime habits are good ones.

The recipes in this chapter are all simple, but interesting enough to hold both your and your toddler's attention. Some can be made in minutes; others are perfect for a day when you have more time. But don't feel like dinner has to be a production. You're cooking for your family after all, not the queen. An omelet with toast and a salad counts as dinner, and a balanced one at that.

no-stress suppers

When you have an active toddler on your hands all day, not to mention work, dinner may be the last thing on your mind... until it's time to eat. Here are a few tricks to ensure that you don't find yourself staring blankly at the fridge at 5:30 pm:

- Make a plan. On Saturday or Sunday jot down what you'll make for dinner each night. Write down a grocery list, and take care of the shopping in one fell swoop.

- Each weekend, prepare at least one dish in large quantities so you can either eat it again later in the week or freeze it for an especially busy night down the road.

- Wash greens and trim vegetables as soon as you bring them home from the grocery store or farmer's market. This cuts down significantly on suppertime prep.

- Don't be afraid to take advantage of convenience foods like rotisserie chicken, peeled and chopped butternut squash, or pre-washed baby spinach if time is tight. You will pay a bit more money for the convenience, but it will still be less expensive (and healthier) than resorting to takeout.

- If you're home, use afternoon naptime to assemble or even cook components for dinner. This is a great time to marinate steak, wash kale, roast squash, mix up a spice rub, or cook a pot of quinoa.

Even if making dinner was a breeze, your stress level can quickly rise if your toddler rejects all or part of the meal. Know that this is completely normal, since many kids get choosier around age two. Follow the feeding strategies on page 158, and stay the course. One strategy that often works for picky eaters is to serve the family meal separated into individual components and allow everyone to assemble their own plates, even if it's just adding on a garnish—or not. Meals where this strategy works especially well feature the Construction Zone icon.

SERVING SIZES

Figuring out the number of servings per recipe is notoriously difficult, especially when you're feeding adults and toddlers at the same meal. The recipes in this chapter make at least four modest, adult and big kid-appropriate servings. But, obviously some grown-ups will eat more (Dad, perhaps?) and toddlers may very well eat less. Just follow your little one's hunger cues, and don't pressure her to eat more than she'd like.

Pineapple
SHRIMP KABOBS

Soak wood or bamboo skewers in water for 30 minutes before grilling so they don't burn, and be sure to remove food from skewers for little ones. To deconstruct this meal, place the marinated ingredients in small bowls and let your kids tell you how they want their kabobs assembled. Or, grill and place the cooked ingredients in separate bowls for your family members to build their own dinners at the table.

1 In a small bowl, whisk together the canola oil, pineapple juice, lime juice, salt, and pepper. Place the shrimp in a dish or zip-top plastic bag. Pour half the marinade over the shrimp. Place the cherry tomatoes and zucchini pieces into another dish or plastic bag, and pour over the remaining marinade. Refrigerate for up to an hour.

2 Thread the shrimp, tomatoes, zucchini, and pineapple chunks onto 8 skewers. Discard any remaining marinade.

3 Heat a grill or grill pan over medium-high heat (or heat a broiler). Grill the kabobs until the shrimp are just opaque, about 2 minutes per side.

Makes 4 servings

¼ CUP CANOLA OIL

¼ CUP PINEAPPLE JUICE

JUICE OF 1 LIME

½ TEASPOON SALT

FRESHLY GROUND PEPPER

1 LB. LARGE SHRIMP, PEELED AND CLEANED

1 CUP CHERRY TOMATOES

½ MEDIUM ZUCCHINI, CUT INTO THICK HALF-MOONS (ABOUT 1 CUP)

8 OZ. PINEAPPLE CUBES (ABOUT 1¾ CUPS)

Nutrition per serving (2 kabob skewers): 256 calories; 16g protein; 15g fat (1g sat. fat); 14g carbohydrates; 2g fiber; 9g sugars; 937mg sodium; 80mg calcium; 1mg iron; 304mg potassium; 42mg Vitamin C; 618IU Vitamin A

SAUCY MEATBALL SLIDERS

1 TEASPOON OLIVE OIL

1 EGG

1 LB. GROUND TURKEY, PREFERABLY 94% LEAN

¼ CUP PANKO

¼ CUP RICOTTA

2 TABLESPOONS CHOPPED PARSLEY

¾ TEASPOON ITALIAN HERB BLEND

¾ TEASPOON SALT

FRESHLY GROUND PEPPER, TO TASTE

1 BATCH GO-TO TOMATO SAUCE (SEE OPPOSITE PAGE), WARMED

12 SLIDER BUNS

Everyone loves a pint-sized sandwich, especially when it's as savory and saucy as these sliders. These meatballs are also crowd pleasers atop pasta.

1 Preheat the oven to 450°F. Grease an 8 x 8 baking dish with the olive oil.

2 Crack the egg into a large bowl, and beat it with a fork. Add the turkey, panko, ricotta, parsley, Italian herb blend, salt, and pepper to taste. Mix with a fork until the ingredients are evenly distributed.

3 Form 12 meatballs and place them in the baking dish in rows, shoulder-to-shoulder in a grid. Bake for 10 minutes.

4 Pour the tomato sauce over the meatballs and bake for an additional 15 minutes or until the temperature on an instant-read thermometer reaches 165°F when inserted into the center of a meatball.

5 To serve, place a meatball and about a tablespoon of sauce on each slider bun.

Makes 12 sliders (6 servings)

MAKE AHEAD: Refrigerate the meatballs and sauce for up to three days. Reheat on the stovetop or in the microwave.

Nutrition per slider: 287 calories; 18g protein; 14g fat (6g sat. fat); 26g carbohydrates; 2g fiber; 8g sugars; 705mg sodium; 102mg calcium; 3mg iron; 445mg potassium; 11mg Vitamin C; 1084IU Vitamin A

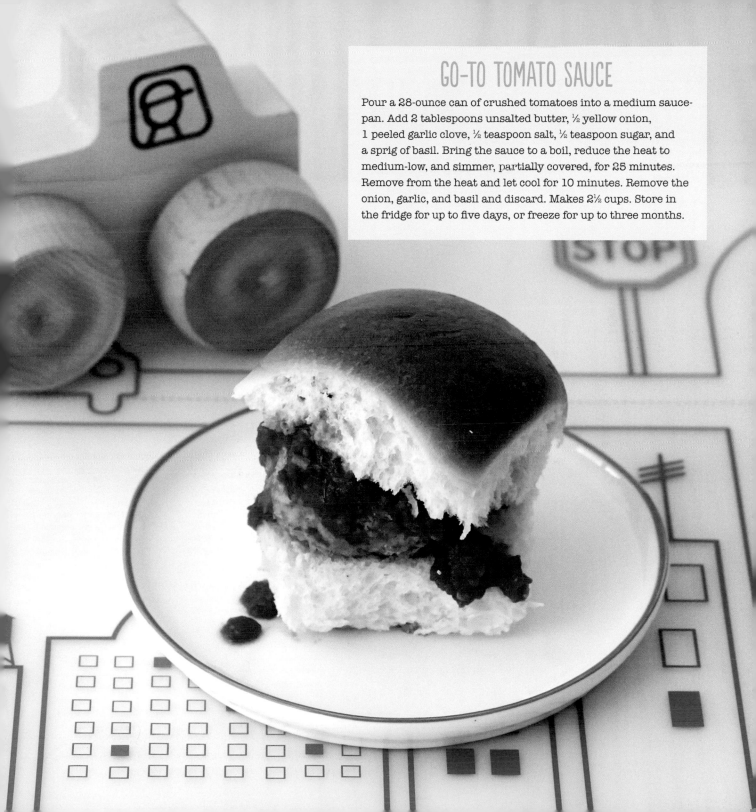

GO-TO TOMATO SAUCE

Pour a 28-ounce can of crushed tomatoes into a medium sauce-pan. Add 2 tablespoons unsalted butter, ½ yellow onion, 1 peeled garlic clove, ½ teaspoon salt, ½ teaspoon sugar, and a sprig of basil. Bring the sauce to a boil, reduce the heat to medium-low, and simmer, partially covered, for 25 minutes. Remove from the heat and let cool for 10 minutes. Remove the onion, garlic, and basil and discard. Makes 2½ cups. Store in the fridge for up to five days, or freeze for up to three months.

FAJITA SALAD

¼ CUP PLUS 2 TABLESPOONS CANOLA OIL, PLUS MORE FOR THE GRILL PAN

2 TABLESPOONS LIME JUICE

3 SCALLIONS, CHOPPED

2 CLOVES GARLIC, CHOPPED

½ TEASPOON CUMIN

½ TEASPOON SALT

1 LB. SKIRT STEAK

PINCH SUGAR

8 CUPS CHOPPED ROMAINE LETTUCE

1 CUP CANNED LOW-SODIUM BLACK BEANS, DRAINED AND RINSED

TORTILLA CHIPS

For serving:
CHOPPED TOMATOES, CHOPPED AVOCADO, SALSA (OPTIONAL)

Fajitas are a favorite at my house, but to get more vegetables into dinner I often nudge them into salad territory. With tortilla chips on the table, no one complains.

1 Put ¼ cup canola oil, the lime juice, scallions, garlic, cumin, and salt into a blender. Blend until smooth. Reserve 2 tablespoons of this marinade and pour the rest into a large zip-top bag. Cut the steak into 3 pieces. Add to the zip-top bag and turn to coat. Marinate in the refrigerator for up to 24 hours. Refrigerate the reserved marinade—this will be the basis of your salad dressing.

2 Heat a grill, grill pan, or large skillet over medium-high heat, and grease with canola oil. Cook the steak until it reaches the desired doneness, 3 to 4 minutes per side for medium, depending on the thickness of the steak. Transfer the steak to a cutting board, cover loosely with foil, and let rest for 5 to 10 minutes.

3 Whisk 2 tablespoons canola oil and a pinch of sugar into the reserved marinade to make the dressing.

4 Slice the steak and serve at the table with the lettuce, beans, tortilla chips, dressing, and any additional toppings.

Makes 4 servings

Nutrition per serving: 551 calories; 30g protein; 36g fat (6g sat. fat); 30g carbohydrates; 6g fiber; 2g sugars; 574mg sodium; 113mg calcium; 5mg iron; 980mg potassium; 9mg Vitamin C; 8316IU Vitamin A

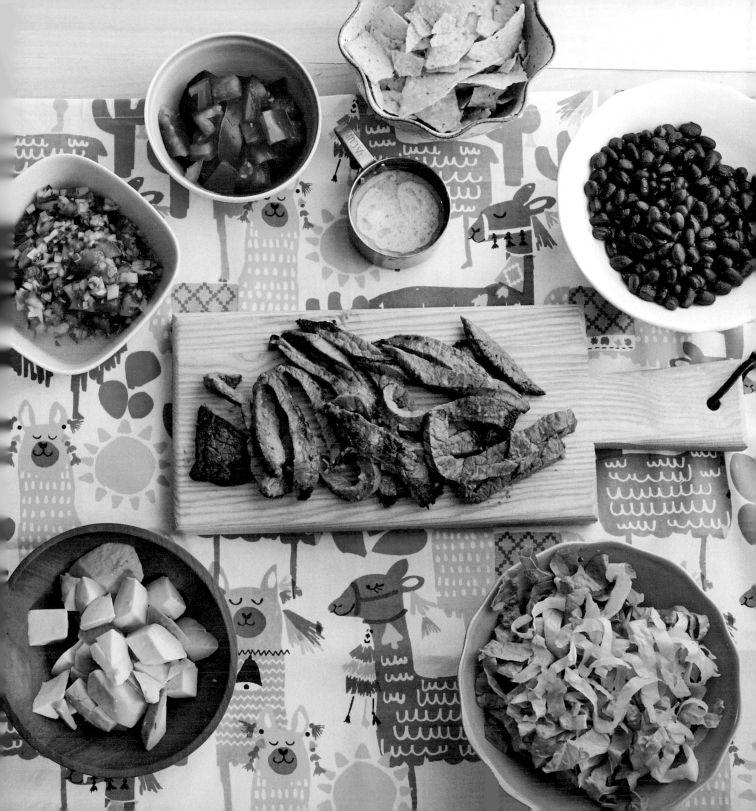

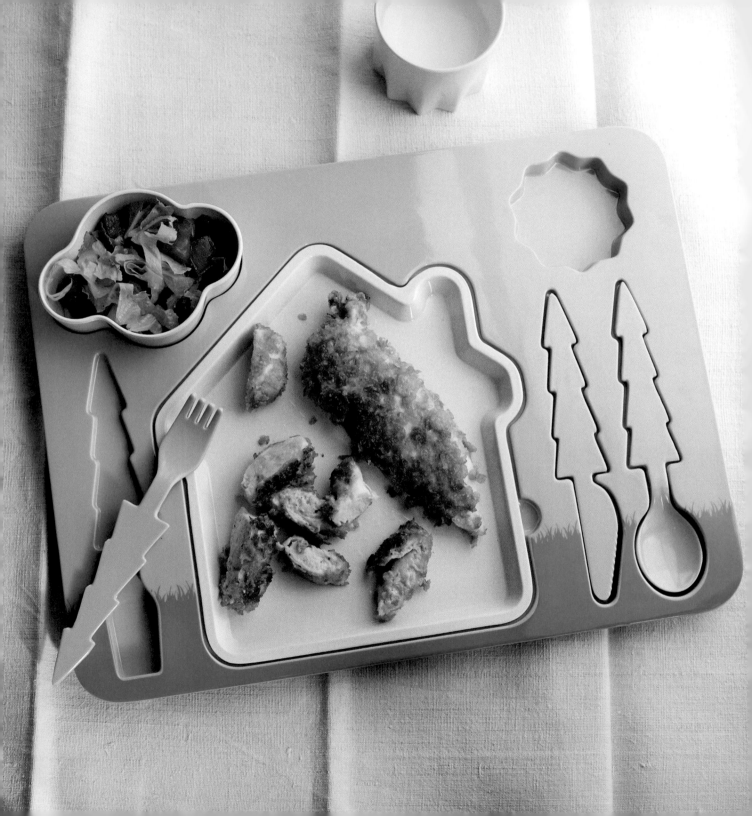

CORNFLAKE CHICKEN CUTLETS

This may be the most indispensible—and versatile—recipe in this book. Everyone from age one to 91 loves a good breaded cutlet. Crushed cornflakes are a tasty coating, but swap in homemade toasted breadcrumbs, panko, pretzel crumbs, crushed saltines, or even popped popcorn you've blitzed in the food processor. And don't stop with chicken. Bread fish fillets, shrimp, veal or pork cutlets, or even wide slices of eggplant for a meal everyone will eat up.

1 LB. CHICKEN CUTLETS

½ TEASPOON SALT

FRESHLY GROUND PEPPER

½ CUP FLOUR

2 EGGS, BEATEN

2 CUPS FINELY CRUSHED CORNFLAKES (ABOUT 4 CUPS WHOLE)

¼ CUP CANOLA OIL

1 Line a rimmed baking sheet with parchment paper. Sprinkle both sides of the chicken cutlets with the salt and pepper.

2 Place the flour in one flat bowl, the eggs in a second, and the cornflakes in a third. Dredge a cutlet in the flour. Shake off excess, and dredge it in the eggs. Finally, dredge the cutlet in the cornflakes. Place on the prepared baking sheet. Repeat with the remaining cutlets.

3 Heat the canola oil in a large skillet over medium-high heat. Add as many cutlets as fit a single layer and cook until golden brown and cooked through, about 3 minutes per side. If the cutlets are browning too quickly, reduce the heat. Don't crowd the pan; cook in batches if necessary to avoid overcrowding. Transfer the cooked cutlets to a cooling rack, and repeat with any remaining cutlets.

Makes 4 servings

Nutrition per serving: 477 calories; 19g protein; 28g fat (5g sat. fat); 36g carbohydrates; 2g fiber; 2g sugars; 923mg sodium; 33mg calcium; 6mg iron; 273mg potassium; 1mg Vitamin C; 682IU Vitamin A

TROPICAL PORK TENDERLOIN

For the pork:

1 TABLESPOON PACKED DARK BROWN SUGAR

2 TEASPOONS CUMIN

1½ TEASPOONS SMOKED PAPRIKA

¾ TEASPOON SALT

3 TABLESPOONS OLIVE OIL

1 LB. PORK TENDERLOIN

For the mango salsa:

1½ CUPS FINELY CHOPPED MANGO (ABOUT 2 MANGOS)

1 SCALLION, CHOPPED

2 TABLESPOONS FINELY CHOPPED RED BELL PEPPER

1 TABLESPOON CHOPPED CILANTRO

PINCH OF SALT

FRESHLY GROUND PEPPER

½ LIME

Get a head start on this dish by stirring together the spice rub earlier in the day. It may seem like only a small step, but you'll feel a mile ahead come dinnertime.

1 In a small bowl, stir together the sugar, cumin, smoked paprika, salt, and 2 tablespoons of olive oil. Cut the pork into 1-inch-thick slices. Flatten the slices with your fingers and rub all over the with spice mixture. Set aside.

2 In a medium bowl, combine the mango, scallion, bell pepper, cilantro, salt, and pepper to taste. Squeeze the lime juice over the salsa.

3 Heat the remaining tablespoon of olive oil in a large skillet over medium-high heat. Cook the pork slices until golden brown on the outside and light pink in the center, 2 to 3 minutes per side. Serve at the table with the mango salsa.

Makes 4 servings

Nutrition per serving: 264 calories; 25g protein; 13g fat (2g sat. fat); 13g carbohydrates; 1g fiber; 11g sugars; 499mg sodium; 18mg calcium; 2mg iron; 597mg potassium; 30mg Vitamin C; 1260IU Vitamin A

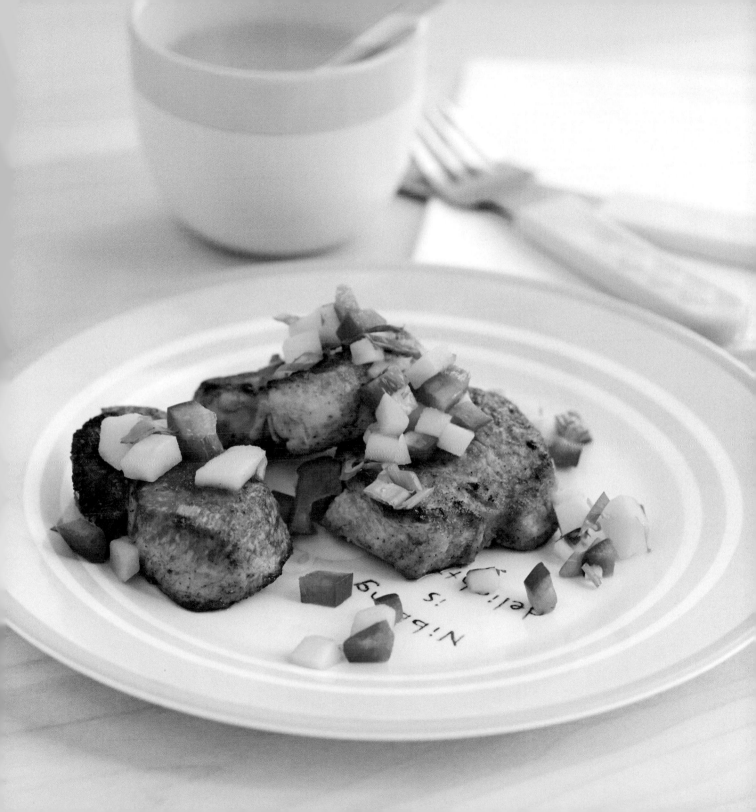

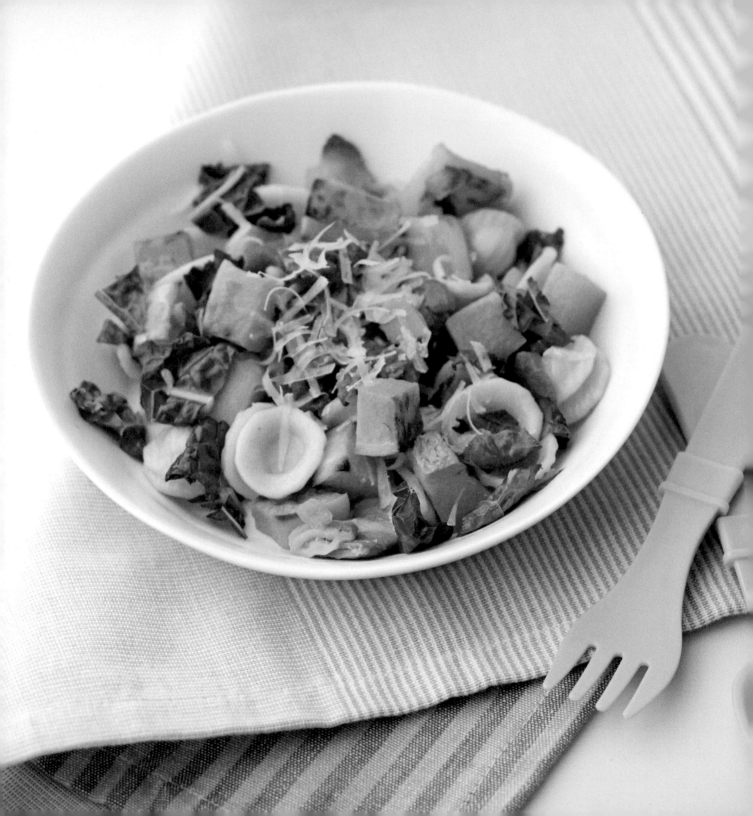

Butternut Squash and
PANCETTA PASTA

You have three main tasks when putting together this hearty, flavorful recipe: roasting the squash, boiling the pasta, and cooking the pancetta and vegetable mixture. Happily they can all happen simultaneously, and whichever components finish first can just hang out and wait for the others. This whole dish comes together in about 35 minutes.

1. Preheat the oven to 425°F. Line a rimmed baking sheet with parchment paper. Toss the butternut squash cubes with a tablespoon of olive oil, ¼ teaspoon salt, and pepper to taste. Spread out on the prepared baking sheet and roast until tender and lightly browned, 25 to 30 minutes.

2. Bring a large pot of salted water to a boil. Cook the pasta according to package directions. Before draining, ladle out 1 cup of cooking water and reserve. Drain the pasta.

3. Heat the remaining tablespoon of olive oil in a large skillet over medium heat. Add the pancetta and onion and cook until the pancetta is lightly browned and the onion is tender, about 10 minutes. Add the kale and the chicken broth. Cook for 5 minutes, scraping up any brown bits at the bottom of the pan.

4. Add the pasta and squash to the skillet along with ½ cup cooking water and ½ teaspoon salt. Stir, adding more cooking water if the pasta seems dry. Transfer to serving bowls and top with grated cheese, if using.

Makes 4 servings

1 LB. BUTTERNUT SQUASH, PEELED AND CUT INTO ¾-INCH CHUNKS

2 TABLESPOONS OLIVE OIL

SALT

FRESHLY GROUND PEPPER, TO TASTE

8 OZ. DRIED ORECCHIETTE PASTA

¼ LB. THICKLY SLICED PANCETTA, DICED

1 CUP CHOPPED YELLOW ONION

4 CUPS SHREDDED TUSCAN KALE (ABOUT ½ BUNCH)

¼ CUP LOW-SODIUM CHICKEN BROTH

GRATED PECORINO OR PARMESAN CHEESE FOR SERVING (OPTIONAL)

Nutrition per serving: 492 calories; 14g protein; 21g fat (5g sat. fat); 66g carbohydrates; 6g fiber; 5g sugars; 712mg sodium; 157mg calcium; 4mg iron; 829mg potassium; 107mg Vitamin C; 22368IU Vitamin A

HONEY MUSTARD CHICKEN

2 TEASPOONS DIJON
MUSTARD

1 TABLESPOON HONEY

3 TABLESPOONS
OLIVE OIL, DIVIDED

2 TABLESPOONS
LEMON JUICE

SALT

1 LB. CHICKEN CUTLETS

FRESHLY GROUND PEPPER

There's no such thing as too many quick and easy chicken recipes. This is a solid, kid-pleasing addition to the repertoire. Marinate the chicken in the morning if you can, but even a 10-minute dip will add flavor. Serve with Roasted Potatoes (see page 212) and a green vegetable like Rosa's Kale Salad (see page 218).

1 In a medium bowl or baking dish, whisk together the mustard, honey, 2 tablespoons olive oil, lemon juice, and ¼ teaspoon salt. Add the chicken cutlets and marinate in the refrigerator for up to 12 hours.

2 Sprinkle each side of the cutlets with salt and pepper. Heat the remaining tablespoon of olive oil in a large skillet over medium-high heat. (Or use a grill pan rubbed with oil.) Sauté the cutlets until browned and cooked through, 2 to 3 minutes per side, cooking in batches if necessary to avoid overcrowding.

Makes 4 servings

COOKING TIP: Make sure the cutlets aren't touching in the pan as they sauté. If they don't have room to breathe they will steam rather than brown and you'll lose out on a lot of flavor.

Nutrition per serving: 373 calories; 15g protein; 26g fat (5g sat. fat); 20g carbohydrates; 1g fiber; 5g sugars; 657mg sodium; 20mg calcium; 1mg iron; 225mg potassium; 4mg Vitamin C; 1IU Vitamin A

SAUSAGE AND PEPPERS

In my experience, bell peppers can be hit or miss with small kids. But simmered with tomatoes and tangled with sausage, they are much more of a sure thing. Be sure to use colorful peppers like red, orange, or yellow, and not the more bitter green variety. Serve over polenta, on pasta, or tucked into rolls.

1 Heat the olive oil in a large skillet. Add the sausage, breaking it into pieces with the back of a spoon. Cook until the sausage is browned, about 5 minutes. Using a slotted spoon, transfer the sausage to a small bowl, leaving the fat in the pan.

2 Add the onion, peppers, salt, and oregano to the pan. Cook over medium heat for 5 minutes. Add the diced tomatoes and their juices. Cover and simmer over medium-low heat, stirring occasionally, for 25 minutes or until the peppers are tender.

3 Return the sausage to the pan and stir to combine. Add freshly ground pepper to taste.

Makes 4 servings

MAKE AHEAD: This dish only gets better if the flavors have a chance to meld overnight in the fridge. Store for up to three days, then reheat in the microwave or on the stovetop in a covered pan.

1 TABLESPOON OLIVE OIL

½ LB. SWEET ITALIAN SAUSAGE, CASINGS REMOVED

1 CUP SLICED ONION (ABOUT ½ ONION)

2 BELL PEPPERS, CORED, SEEDED, AND THINLY SLICED

½ TEASPOON SALT

1 TEASPOON DRIED OREGANO

1¼ CUPS DICED TOMATOES WITH JUICES (FROM A 14.5-OZ. CAN)

FRESHLY GROUND PEPPER, TO TASTE

Nutrition per serving: 164 calories; 11g protein; 8g fat (2g sat. fat); 13g carbohydrates; 3g fiber; 6g sugars; 794mg sodium; 51mg calcium; 1mg iron; 477mg potassium; 63mg Vitamin C; 360IU Vitamin A

COCONUT CURRY MUSSELS

1 CUP CANNED LIGHT COCONUT MILK

½ CUP CANNED DICED TOMATOES WITH JUICES

2 TEASPOONS LIME JUICE

2 TEASPOONS BROWN SUGAR

1 TEASPOON FISH SAUCE

½ TEASPOON GRATED FRESH GINGER

¼ TEASPOON THAI RED CURRY PASTE, OR TO TASTE

2 LBS. MUSSELS, DEBEARDED IF NECESSARY AND RINSED

2 TABLESPOONS CHOPPED CILANTRO

This may sound shocking, but I believe that mussels are the ultimate kid-friendly food. How fun is it to scoop your dinner out of seashells? Mom and dad also like them because they're high in protein and iron and quite inexpensive. Most mussels for sale these days have already been debearded, but if they haven't, ask the person at the fish counter to do it for you. Before cooking, discard any open mussels that won't stay closed with a tap. Serve with a green salad and bread for soaking up the sauce.

1 Put the coconut milk, tomatoes, lime juice, brown sugar, fish sauce, grated ginger, and curry paste in a large wide-bottomed pot. Whisk, then bring to a simmer over medium heat. Simmer for 5 minutes. Taste the broth to see if it needs more sour (lime juice), salt (fish sauce), or sweet (brown sugar): you want a nice balance.

2 Add the mussels. Cover the pot, reduce the heat to medium-low, and cook until the mussels have opened, 5 to 10 minutes. Transfer the mussels to serving dishes, discarding any that failed to open. Ladle the sauce over top and sprinkle with cilantro.

Makes 4 servings

Nutrition per serving: 334 calories; 27g protein; 17g fat (5g sat. fat); 17g carbohydrates; 1g fiber; 4g sugars; 858mg sodium; 71mg calcium; 10mg iron; 825mg potassium; 25mg Vitamin C; 453IU Vitamin A

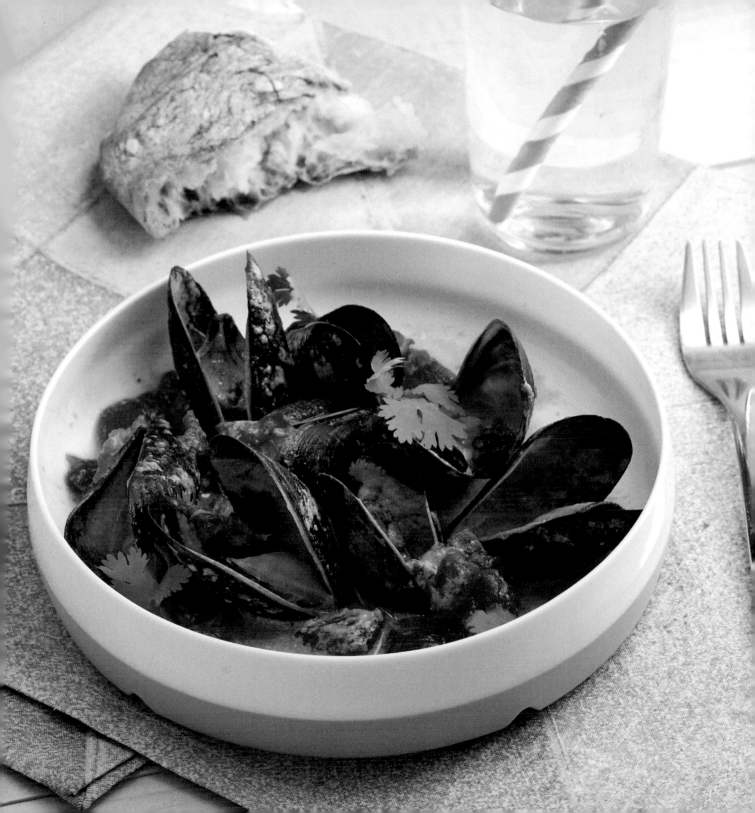

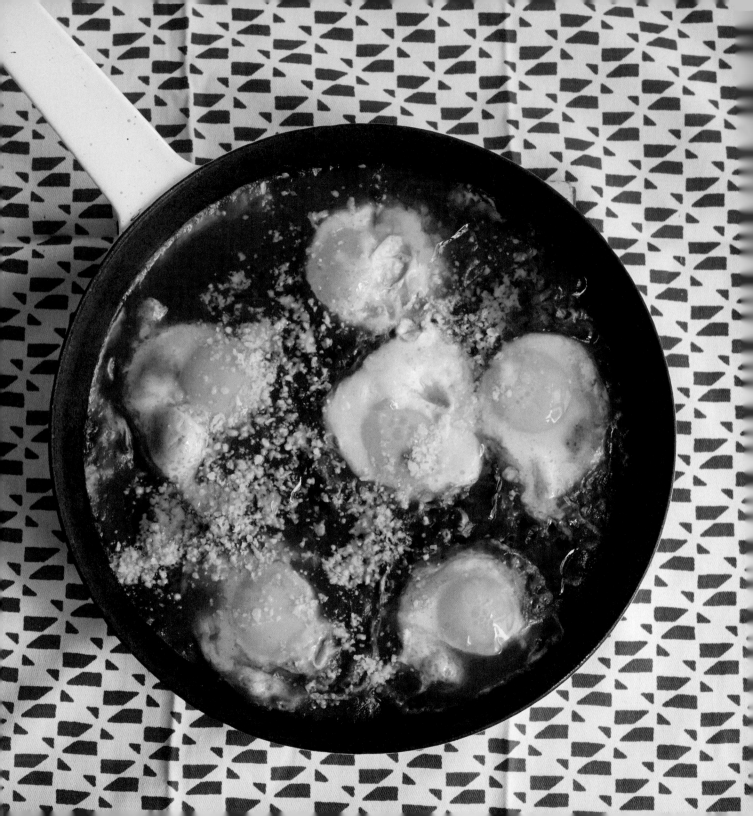

EGGS IN PURGATORY

Served with bread and salad, this is the ultimate quick weeknight meal. The only requirement is that you have tomato sauce on hand. Homemade sauce doesn't take long to prepare, but I'll look the other way if you use a jarred marinara. Make two eggs for big kids and grown-ups and one for toddlers.

2 CUPS GO-TO TOMATO SAUCE (SEE PAGE 191)

6 EGGS

1 TEASPOON OLIVE OIL

GRATED PARMESAN CHEESE, TO TASTE

1 In a 10-inch skillet, bring the tomato sauce to a simmer. Crack the eggs onto the sauce. Cover and cook on medium-low until the whites have firmed up, 8 to 10 minutes.

2 Transfer the eggs and sauce to serving dishes. Drizzle with olive oil and sprinkle with grated Parmesan cheese.

Makes 4 servings

Nutrition per serving (1 egg and ⅓ cup sauce): 205 calories; 11g protein; 13g fat (5g sat. fat); 14g carbohydrates; 3g fiber; 8g sugars; 543mg sodium; 100mg calcium; 3mg iron; 577mg potassium; 16mg Vitamin C; 1612IU Vitamin A

ASIAN PORK LETTUCE WRAPS

Sesame-Soy Dipping Sauce:

2 TABLESPOONS REDUCED-SODIUM SOY SAUCE

1 TABLESPOON SESAME OIL

1 TABLESPOON WATER

1 TEASPOON RICE VINEGAR

½ TEASPOON HONEY

Pork:

1 LB. GROUND PORK

¼ TEASPOON SALT

1 SCALLION

1 TEASPOON GRATED GINGER

1 CLOVE GARLIC, CHOPPED

¼ CUP FINELY CHOPPED WATER CHESTNUTS

1 TABLESPOON SOY SAUCE

For serving:

BIBB (BOSTON) LETTUCE LEAVES, CARROT STRIPS, CILANTRO, MINT LEAVES

This meal is a stellar example of a deconstructed dinner. You have your meat, your various veg, and a sauce. Everyone decides how much of each component he or she would like.

1 **To make the sauce:** Stir together 2 tablespoons soy sauce, the sesame oil, water, rice vinegar, and honey.

2 Brown the pork in a large skillet over medium-high heat. Sprinkle with the salt and cook until no longer pink. Drain and discard the fat. Return the pork to the pan.

3 Add the scallion, ginger, garlic, water chestnuts, and 1 tablespoon soy sauce, and cook over medium-low heat until the ginger and garlic are fragrant, about 2 minutes.

4 Serve on lettuce leaves with carrot strips, cilantro sprigs, and mint leaves, and the sesame-soy sauce for dipping.

Makes 4 servings

Nutrition per serving: 351 calories; 20g protein; 27g fat (9g sat. fat); 4g carbohydrates; 0g fiber; 2g sugars; 686mg sodium; 19mg calcium; 1mg iron; 380mg potassium; 1mg Vitamin C; 8IU Vitamin A

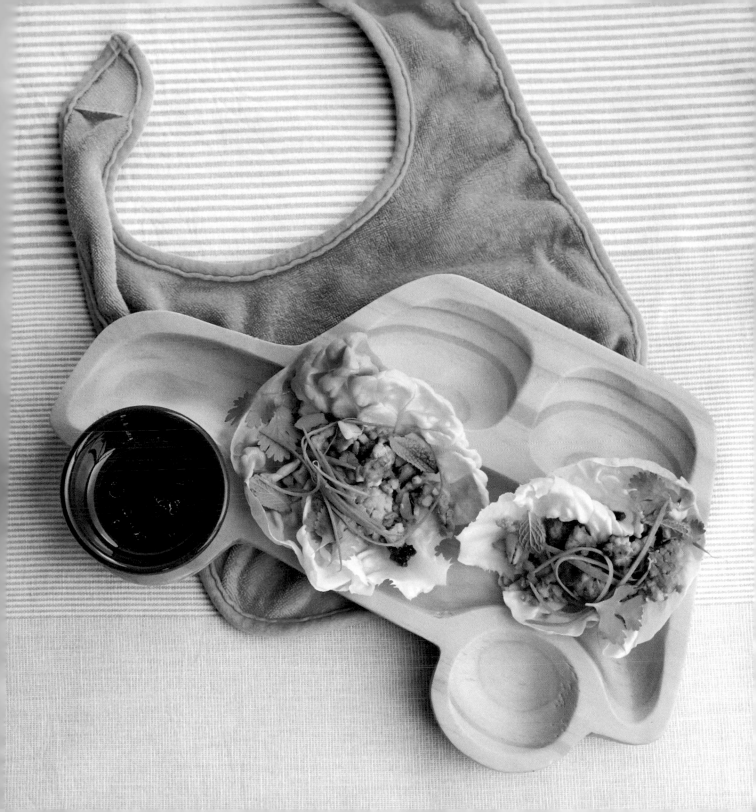

CROWD-PLEASING CHILI

1 LB. 85% LEAN
GROUND BEEF

1 CUP CHOPPED ONION

1 CLOVE GARLIC, MINCED

ONE 28-OZ. CAN DICED
TOMATOES

ONE 15-OZ. CAN LOW-
SODIUM PINTO BEANS,
DRAINED AND RINSED

2 PLUM TOMATOES, CHOPPED

¼ CUP KETCHUP

1 TEASPOON CHILI POWDER

¾ TEASPOON GROUND CUMIN

¾ TEASPOON SALT

⅛ TEASPOON CINNAMON

FRESHLY GROUND PEPPER

For serving (optional):
SHREDDED CHEDDAR CHEESE,
CHOPPED SCALLIONS,
DICED AVOCADO

I grew up with a version of this mild, thick chili, and as kids we were always happy to see it on the table. This is a perfect candidate to double. Save half for later in the week or stash it in the freezer.

1 Put the ground beef, onion, and garlic in a large pot over medium heat. Sauté until the beef is no longer pink, breaking it up with a spoon. Drain, discard the fat, and return to the pot.

2 Add the diced tomatoes, pinto beans, plum tomatoes, ketchup, chili powder, cumin, salt, and cinnamon. Bring to a boil, then reduce the heat so the chili simmers. Cover and cook for an hour, stirring occasionally. Add freshly ground pepper to taste.

3 Divide the chili between bowls and serve with the shredded cheese, chopped scallions, and/or diced avocado at the table.

Makes 4 servings

MAKE AHEAD: Keep in the fridge for up to three days. Reheat in the microwave or on the stovetop.

Nutrition per serving: 398 calories; 28g protein; 18g fat (7g sat. fat); 32g carbohydrates; 5g fiber; 12g sugars; 729mg sodium; 109mg calcium; 4mg iron; 691mg potassium; 24mg Vitamin C; 1387IU Vitamin A

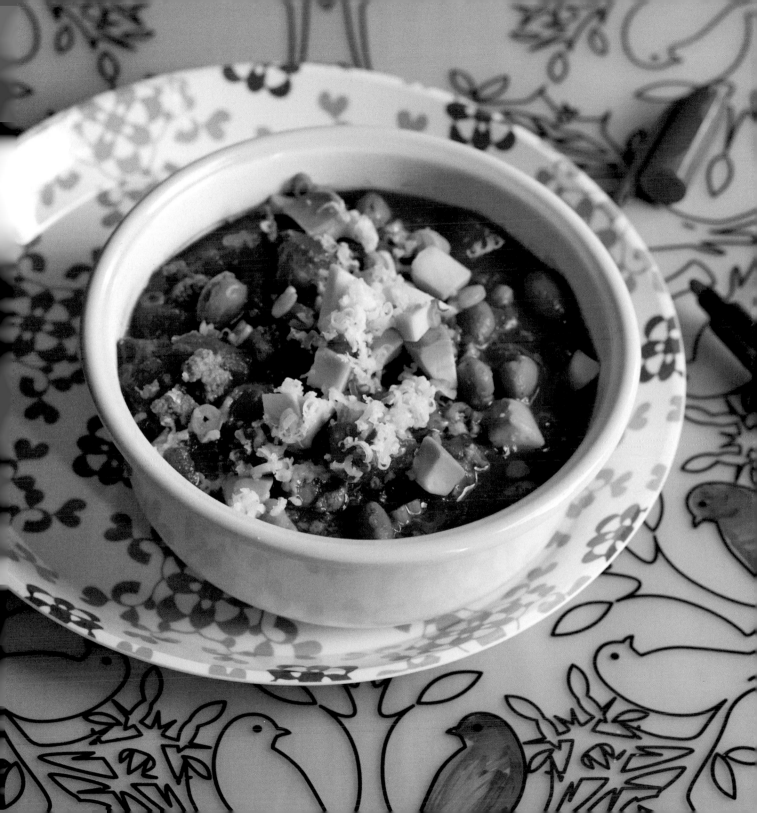

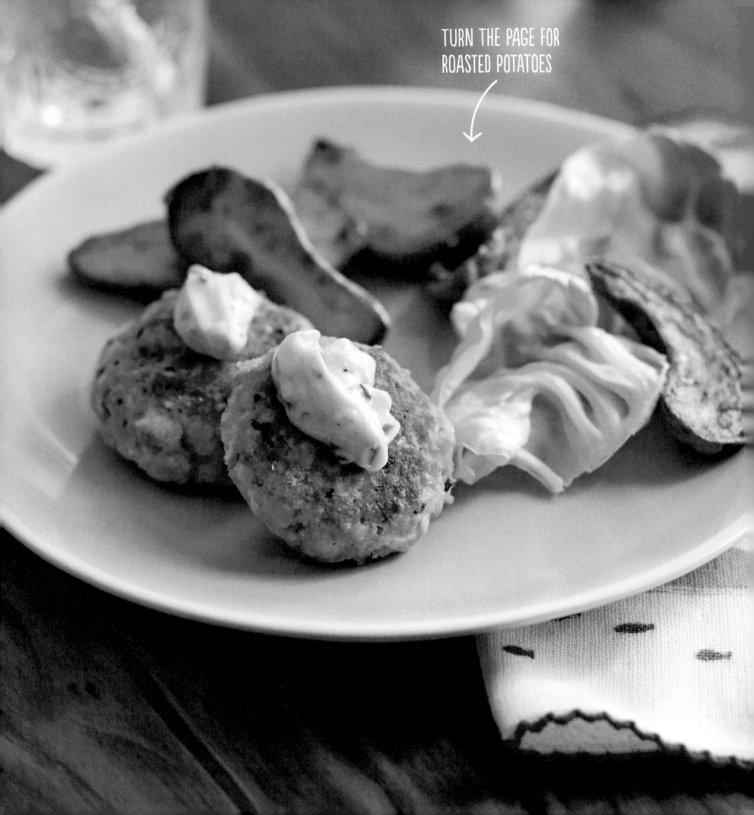

TURN THE PAGE FOR
ROASTED POTATOES

SALMON CAKES
with Garlic Mayo

This is the tastiest way I know to get salmon into kids (and grown-ups). Wrap these small patties in lettuce leaves, serve on slider buns, or just let kids eat them with their hands.

1 In a small bowl, stir together the mayonnaise, mustard, chives, garlic, and pepper to taste.

2 Pulse the salmon in a food processor until finely chopped. Transfer to a medium bowl. Add ¼ cup of the mayonnaise mixture, the panko, salt, and pepper to taste. Mix just until combined, and form into 8 small patties. Add the lemon juice to the remaining mayonnaise mixture and stir to combine.

3 Heat the olive oil in a large skillet over medium heat. Sauté the patties until golden brown, 2 to 3 minutes per side. Serve with the mayonnaise mixture.

Makes 4 servings

MAKE AHEAD: Complete the recipe through Step 2. Refrigerate the patties and mayo mixture for up to 24 hours. Cook as directed in Step 3. You can also freeze the assembled patties for up to three months. Defrost overnight in the fridge and cook as directed.

½ CUP MAYONNAISE

2 TEASPOONS DIJON MUSTARD

2 TABLESPOONS FINELY CHOPPED CHIVES

1 CLOVE GARLIC, MINCED

FRESHLY GROUND PEPPER, TO TASTE

1 LB. SALMON FILLETS (PREFERABLY WILD), SKIN REMOVED, CUT INTO CHUNKS

¼ CUP PANKO

½ TEASPOON SALT

1 TEASPOON LEMON JUICE

2 TABLESPOONS OLIVE OIL

Nutrition per serving (2 patties): 432 calories; 23g protein; 34g fat (5g sat. fat); 6g carbohydrates; 0g fiber; 1g sugars; 630mg sodium; 29mg calcium; 1mg iron; 578mg potassium; 2mg Vitamin C; 110IU Vitamin A

ROASTED POTATOES

1 LB. FINGERLING POTATOES, HALVED LENGTHWISE

1 TABLESPOON OLIVE OIL

1 TABLESPOON CHOPPED SAGE

¼ TEASPOON SALT, PLUS MORE TO TASTE

FRESHLY GROUND PEPPER, TO TASTE

Think of roasted vegetables as your suppertime secret weapon. Simply toss some veggies with olive oil, salt, and pepper, put them in the oven, and then forget about them while you make the rest of the meal. Browned, crispy roasted veggies are often more appealing than their steamed or sautéed counterparts.

Use this same method for sweet potato chunks, broccoli or cauliflower florets, carrot sticks, or halved Brussels sprouts. Just omit or switch up the herb and adjust the roasting time as necessary.

1 Preheat the oven to 425°F. Line a rimmed baking sheet with parchment paper. Toss the potatoes with the olive oil, sage, salt, and pepper to taste. Lay cut-side down on the parchment paper.

2 Roast until golden brown, about 40 minutes. Sprinkle with more salt to taste.

Makes 4 servings

Nutrition per serving: 116 calories; 2g protein; 4g fat (1g sat. fat); 20g carbohydrates; 3g fiber; 1g sugars; 152mg sodium; 13mg calcium; 1mg iron; 472mg potassium; 22mg Vitamin C; 2IU Vitamin A

FARROTTO *with* PESTO AND CHICKEN SAUSAGE

Farro is a nutty, chewy whole grain that is a staple in Italy and becoming more widely available. Use it in salads like you would barley or quinoa or as a bed for meat or vegetables. It also makes a terrific risotto-like dish with minimal stirring. You may not use all of the stock the recipe calls for. Once the farro is tender, but not yet mushy, it's ready.

2 CUPS SEMI-PEARLED FARRO

5 CUPS LOW-SODIUM CHICKEN STOCK

2 TEASPOONS OLIVE OIL

6 OZ. FULLY COOKED CHICKEN SAUSAGE, SUCH AS AIDELLS, HALVED LENGTHWISE AND SLICED

⅓ CUP PESTO OR SPINACH PESTO (SEE PAGE 105)

1 Place the farro and 2 cups chicken stock in a medium saucepan. Bring to a boil. Reduce the heat to medium and simmer until most of the stock is below the level of the farro. Add more stock ½ cup at a time and continue simmering until the farro is tender, but not mushy. This should take 4 to 5 cups of stock and about 30 minutes.

2 While the farro is cooking, heat the olive oil in a medium skillet over medium heat. Add the sausage and cook until browned, about 5 minutes.

3 Stir the pesto into the farro. Divide between serving bowls and top with the browned sausage.

Makes 4 servings

Nutrition per serving: 625 calories; 29g protein; 20g fat (2g sat. fat); 79g carbohydrates; 15g fiber; 0g sugars; 509mg sodium; 72mg calcium; 7mg iron; 258mg potassium; 1mg Vitamin C; 50IU Vitamin A

CHICKEN SOBA SOUP

6 CUPS LOW-SODIUM
CHICKEN BROTH

2 CLOVES GARLIC,
THINLY SLICED

1-INCH PIECE FRESH
GINGER, PEELED AND CUT
INTO THIN MATCHSTICKS

1 BONELESS, SKINLESS
CHICKEN BREAST

6 OZ. SOBA NOODLES

¼ TEASPOON SALT

1 MEDIUM HEAD BABY BOK
CHOY, CHOPPED, STEMS AND
LEAVES SEPARATED

1 TEASPOON LEMON JUICE

2 SCALLIONS, CHOPPED

Soba noodles add a fun factor to this Asian version of chicken noodle soup. Save any extra for lunch the next day.

1 In a large pot, bring the chicken broth, garlic, and ginger to a boil. Add the chicken breast. Reduce the heat to a bare simmer, cover, and poach the chicken until cooked through, 15 to 20 minutes. Transfer the chicken to a plate to cool a bit, then shred or chop it into bite-sized pieces.

2 Bring the chicken broth to a boil. Add the soba noodles, salt, and bok choy stem pieces. Cook for 4 minutes or until the noodles are tender. Take the pan off the heat. Add the bok choy leaves, lemon juice, and the chicken. Divide between bowls and serve with the scallions at the table.

Makes 4 generous servings

MAKE AHEAD: Refrigerate overnight and reheat on the stovetop or in the microwave.

Nutrition per serving: 276 calories; 26g protein; 4g fat (1g sat. fat); 38g carbohydrates; 0g fiber; 1g sugars; 677mg sodium; 60mg calcium; 2mg iron; 712mg potassium; 13mg Vitamin C; 1130IU Vitamin A

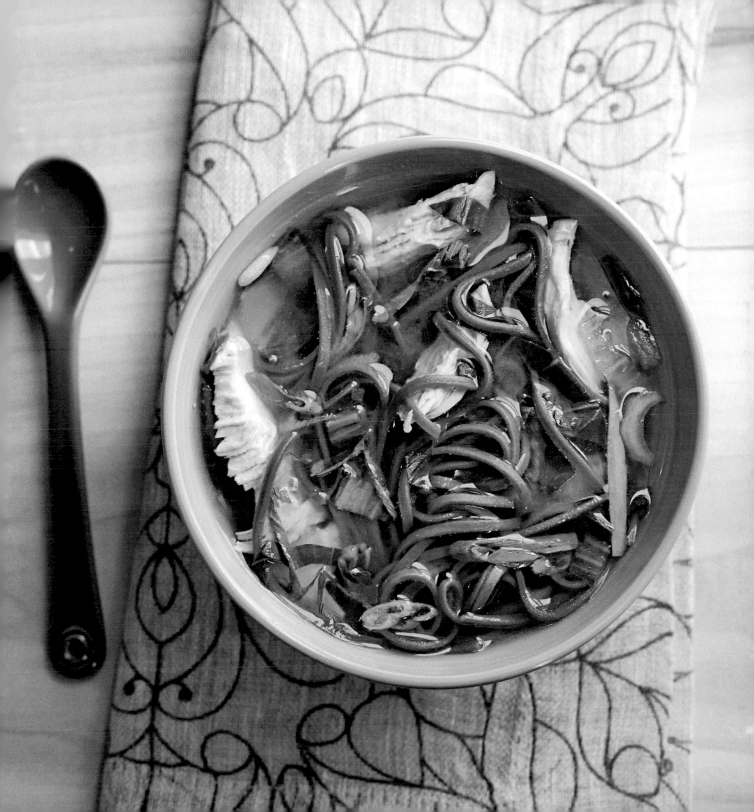

LAMB-OLIVE BURGERS

1 LB. GROUND LAMB

½ CUP PITTED OLIVES, SUCH AS KALAMATA, CHOPPED

1 CLOVE GARLIC, FINELY CHOPPED

½ TEASPOON SALT

FRESHLY GROUND PEPPER, TO TASTE

1 TEASPOON CANOLA OIL

4 WHOLE-WHEAT HAMBURGER BUNS, TOASTED

To deconstruct this meal, shape one burger before adding the olives, and then serve the olives on the side to your toddler. My favorite accompaniments are sweet potato fries and a spinach salad.

1 In a large bowl, mix together the lamb, olives, garlic, salt, and pepper to taste. I find that my hands are the best tools for this job. Shape the mixture into 4 to 6 patties, depending on the age of your eaters.

2 Rub a grill pan or large skillet with the canola oil and heat over medium-high heat. Cook the burgers to desired doneness, about 4 minutes per side for medium-well. Serve on the toasted buns.

Makes 4 servings

COOKING TIP: Use your thumb to make an indentation in the center of each burger. This will help the patty cook more evenly.

WHOLESOME TIP

The USDA recommends all ground meat hit 165°F when tested with an instant-read thermometer; this is considered "well done." At my house we tend to serve burgers pink in the middle, so on the medium to medium-well end of the spectrum, but make your own choice.

Nutrition per serving: 456 calories; 22g protein; 31g fat (12g sat. fat); 22g carbohydrates; 0g fiber; 0g sugars; 664mg sodium; 31mg calcium; 2mg iron; 256mg potassium; 0mg Vitamin C; 53IU Vitamin A

MOROCCAN BEEF STEW

Tender stews are an ideal dish for grown-ups and toddlers to share. This recipe makes enough for two dinners, so you can freeze half for later.

1 Cut the beef into 1½-inch chunks. In a large bowl, toss with ½ teaspoon salt, pepper, and the flour.

2 Heat 2 tablespoons of olive oil in a large pot or Dutch oven over medium-high heat. Brown the meat on all sides, cooking in batches if necessary to avoid overcrowding, about 8 minutes total per batch. Transfer the meat to a bowl.

3 Add 1 tablespoon of olive oil to the pot and turn the heat to medium-low. Add the onion and cook until nearly tender, about 6 minutes. Add the cumin and cinnamon and cook for another minute. Add the tomato paste and cook for 2 more minutes, stirring frequently.

4 Add the broth, raise the heat to high, and bring to a boil, scraping up any browned bits from the bottom of the pan. Return the meat and any juices to the pan. Reduce the heat to medium-low, cover, and simmer for 1 hour.

5 Peel the carrots and slice into half-moons, rinse and drain the chickpeas, and slice the prunes in half. Just before using, peel the potatoes and chop them into 1-inch chunks.

6 Add the carrots, chickpeas, prunes, potatoes, and 1 teaspoon salt to the pot. Simmer, partially covered, for 45 minutes or until the meat and vegetables are tender. Stir in the cilantro.

Makes 8 servings

2 LBS. BEEF STEW MEAT

1½ TEASPOONS SALT

FRESHLY GROUND PEPPER

2 TABLESPOONS FLOUR

3 TABLESPOONS OLIVE OIL

1 CUP CHOPPED ONION

4 TEASPOONS CUMIN

1 TEASPOON CINNAMON

2 TABLESPOONS TOMATO PASTE

6 CUPS LOW-SODIUM BEEF BROTH

3 CARROTS

ONE 15-OZ. CAN LOW-SODIUM CHICKPEAS

1 CUP PITTED PRUNES

1½ LBS. RED POTATOES

½ CUP CHOPPED CILANTRO

Nutrition per serving: 388 calories; 31g protein; 11g fat (3g sat. fat); 43g carbohydrates; 5g fiber; 12g sugars; 956mg sodium; 62mg calcium; 4mg iron; 1134mg potassium; 11mg Vitamin C; 2925IU Vitamin A

ROSA'S KALE SALAD

1 BUNCH TUSCAN KALE, THICK STEMS REMOVED, SLICED INTO RIBBONS (ABOUT 10 CUPS)

2 TABLESPOONS OLIVE OIL

1 TEASPOON LEMON JUICE

¼ TEASPOON SALT, PLUS MORE TO TASTE

FRESHLY GROUND PEPPER, TO TASTE

1 CLOVE GARLIC, MINCED

3 TABLESPOONS PARMESAN CHEESE, PLUS MORE TO TASTE

My daughter piles huge quantities of this salad on her plate, and requests it in her lunchbox. Don't skimp on the salt or Parmesan cheese. Your job here is to make this salad taste AWESOME.

1 Place the kale ribbons in a large bowl. Add the olive oil, lemon juice, ¼ teaspoon salt, and pepper to taste. Using tongs or your hands, mix well, making sure the olive oil is rubbed into the kale leaves.

2 Add the garlic and Parmesan cheese and toss again. Taste for seasoning, adding more salt, pepper, and Parmesan if necessary. You don't want to taste the bitterness of the kale.

Makes 4 servings

MAKE AHEAD: This is a rare salad that keeps well in the fridge. Store it for up to two days.

Nutrition per serving: 143 calories; 6g protein; 8g fat (2g sat. fat); 15g carbohydrates; 3g fiber; 6g sugars; 244mg sodium; 239mg calcium; 3mg iron; 673mg potassium; 179mg Vitamin C; 22922IU Vitamin A

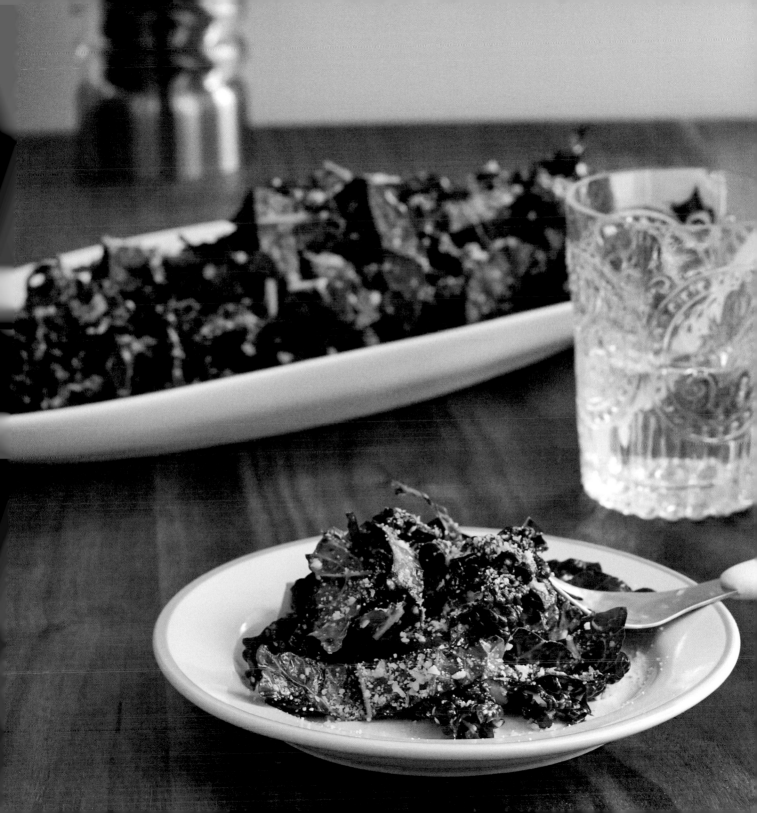

metric conversion guide

Note: The recipes in this cookbook have not been developed or tested using metric measures.
When converting recipes to metric, some variations in quality may be noted.

VOLUME

U.S. Units	Canadian Metric	Australian Metric
¼ teaspoon	1 mL	1 ml
½ teaspoon	2 mL	2 ml
1 teaspoon	5 mL	5 ml
1 tablespoon	15 mL	20 ml
¼ cup	50 mL	60 ml
⅓ cup	75 mL	80 ml
½ cup	125 mL	125 ml
⅔ cup	150 mL	170 ml
¾ cup	175 mL	190 ml
1 cup	250 mL	250 ml
1 quart	1 liter	1 liter
1 ½ quarts	1.5 liters	1.5 liters
2 quarts	2 liters	2 liters
2 ½ quarts	2.5 liters	2.5 liters
3 quarts	3 liters	3 liters
4 quarts	4 liters	4 liters

WEIGHT

U.S. Units	Canadian Metric	Australian Metric
1 ounce	30 grams	30 grams
2 ounces	55 grams	60 grams
3 ounces	85 grams	90 grams
4 ounces (¼ pound)	115 grams	125 grams
8 ounces (½ pound)	225 grams	225 grams
16 ounces (1 pound)	455 grams	500 grams
1 pound	455 grams	0.5 kilograms

MEASUREMENTS

Inches	Centimeters
1	2.5
2	5.0
3	7.5
4	10.0
5	12.5
6	15.0
7	17.5
8	20.5
9	23.0
10	25.5
11	28.0
12	30.5
13	33.0

TEMPERATURES

Fahrenheit	Celsius
32°	0°
212°	100°
250°	120°
275°	140°
300°	150°
325°	160°
350°	180°
375°	190°
400°	200°
425°	220°
450°	230°
475°	240°
500°	260°

index

Page numbers in *italic* indicate photos

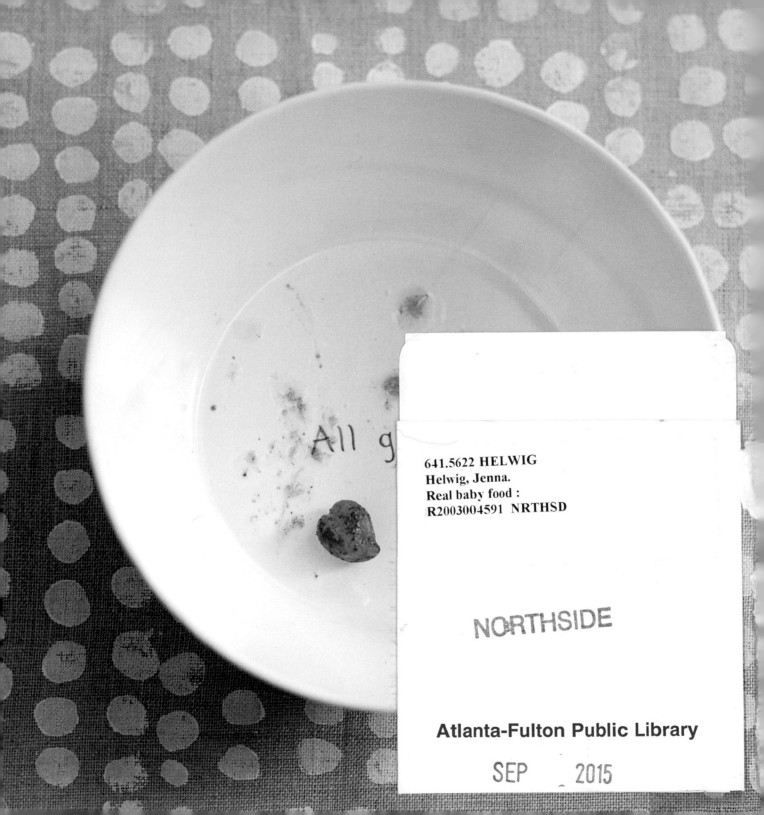

All g